PCOS DIET COOKBOOK

The Complete Guide with Flavorful Recipes to
Manage Polycystic Ovary Syndrome,
Regulate your Hormones and improve Fertility

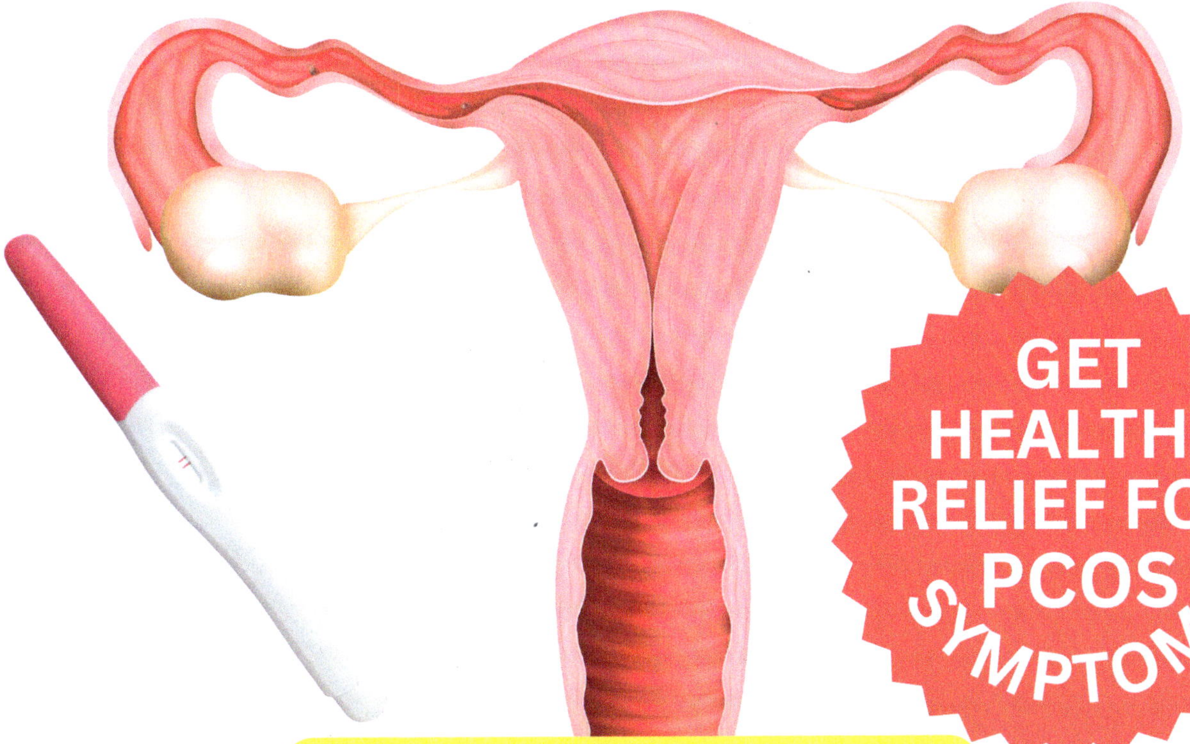

GET HEALTHY RELIEF FOR PCOS SYMPTOMS

EMILY LEXIE

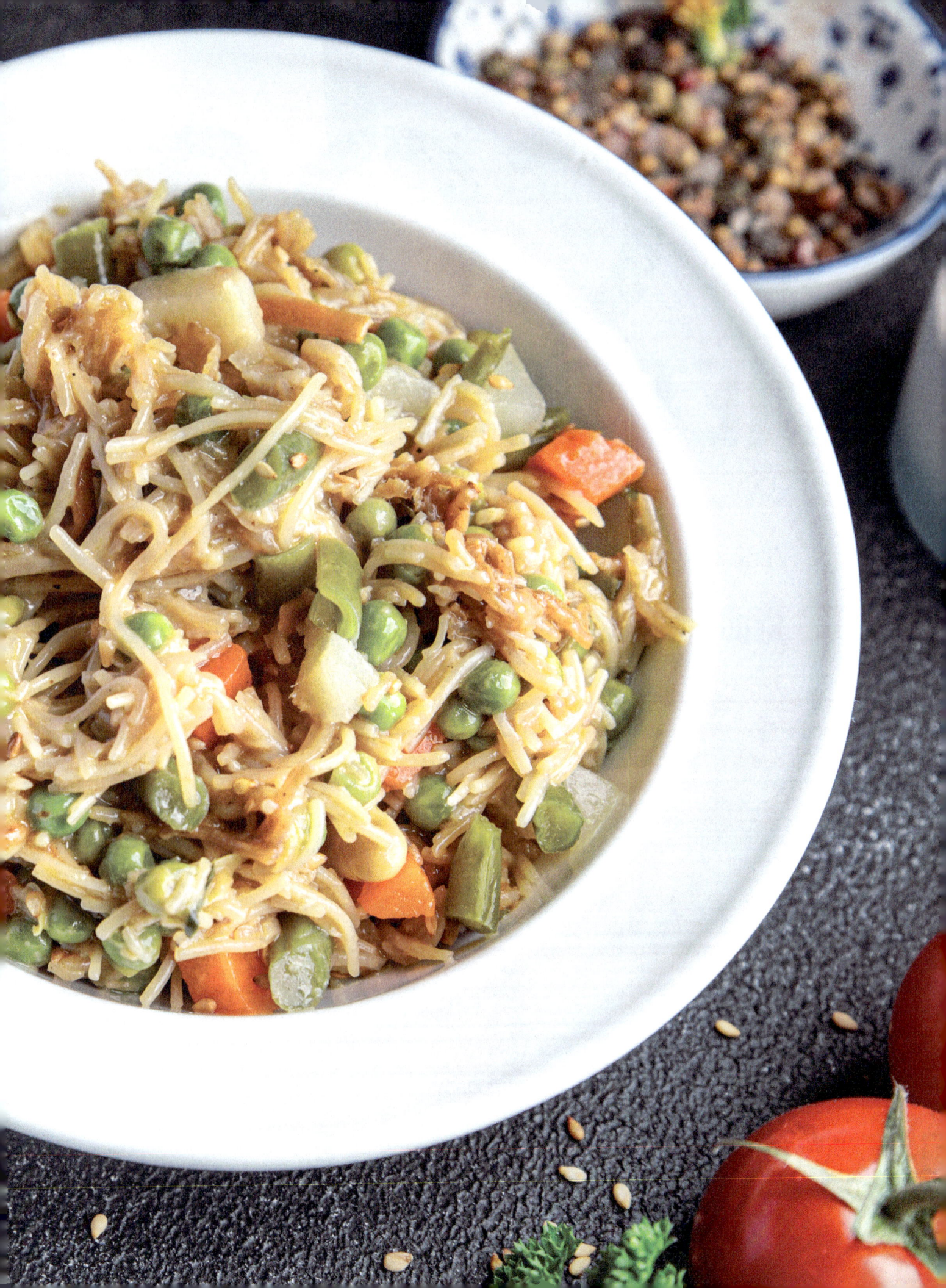

Copyright © 2024 by Emily Lexie
All rights reserved.

No part of this publication may be reproduced, distributed, or transmitted in any form or by any means, including photocopying, recording, or other electronic or mechanical methods, without the prior written permission of the author, except in the case of brief quotations embodied in critical reviews and certain other noncommercial uses permitted by copyright law

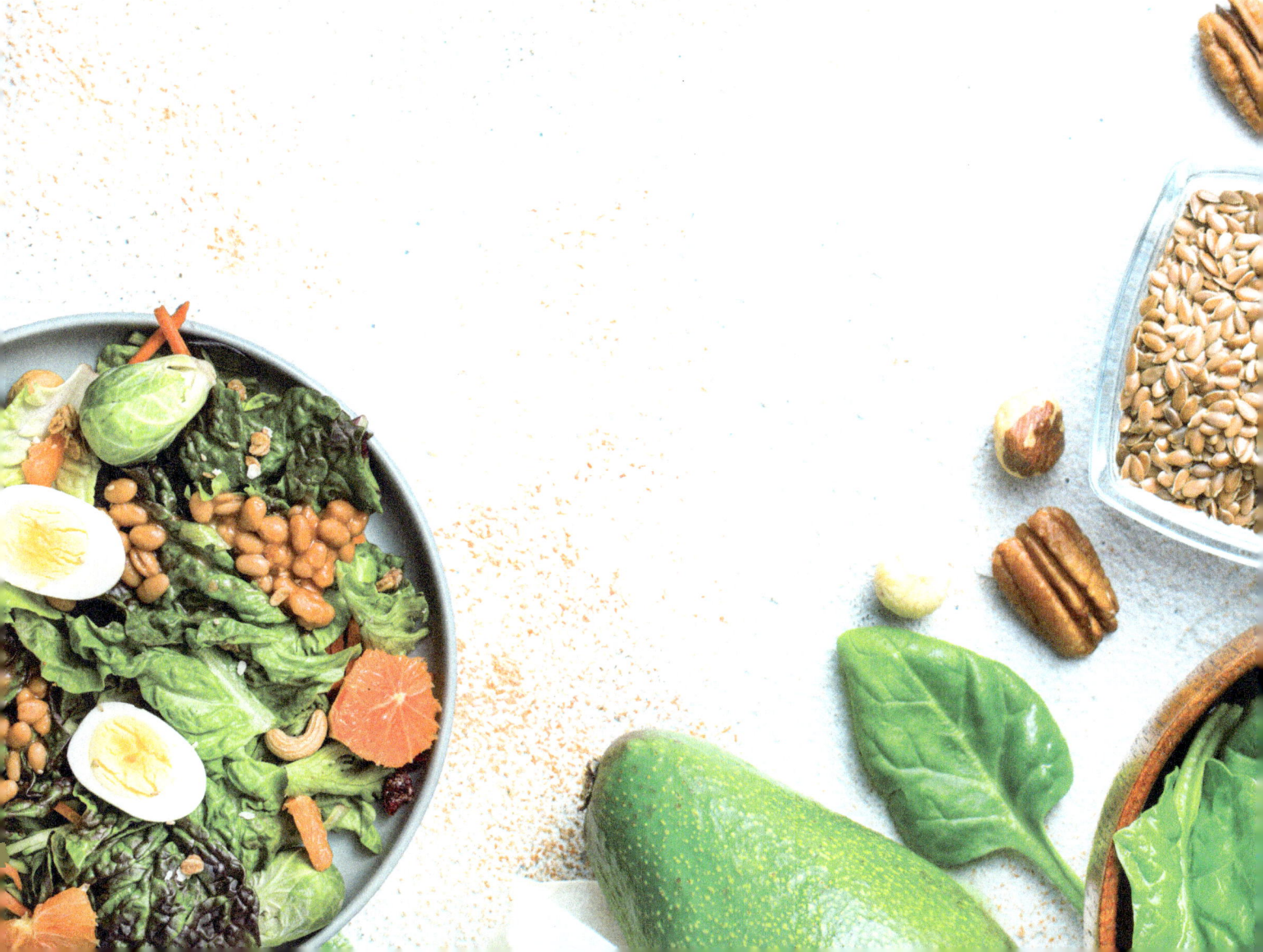

Expressing my heartfelt gratitude

I am deeply grateful for your decision to purchase this Cookbook tailored specifically for women managing PCOS symptoms. I'm thrilled to hear about your experience with these recipes and how they've positively impacted your health journey

As an independent publisher, your voice and feedback hold immense value. They not only inspire me to continually refine my work but also guide others on their path toward being able to balance their hormones and manage their PCOS symptoms as well. If you found value in this Diet Cookbook, I kindly request that you consider leaving a review on Amazon.

Your insights and experiences can make a profound difference in both supporting my mission and assisting countless others in benefiting from this Cookbook.

From the depths of my heart, I extend my sincere gratitude for joining me on this journey. Your support fuels my passion and purpose.

With warm regards,

Emily Lexie

PCOS DIET COOKBOOK

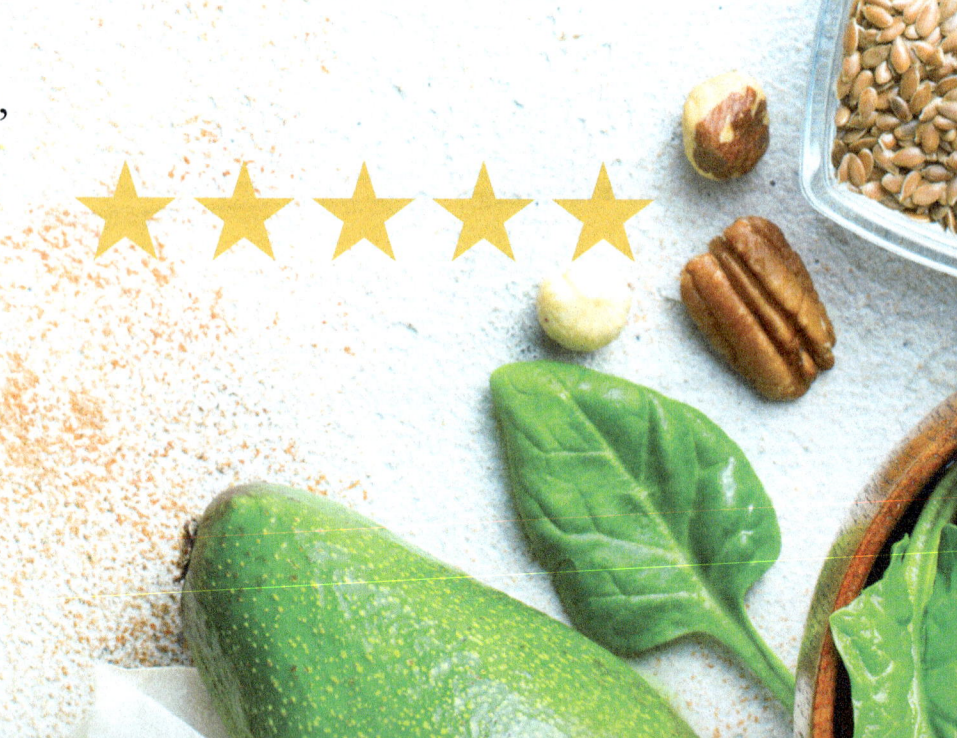

TABLE OF CONTENT

Introduction — 7

Chapter 1: Understanding PCOS — 9-12
- What is PCOS?
- Causes of PCOS
- Symptoms and Diagnosis
- Treatment Options
- The role of diet in managing PCOS
- Impact of PCOS on fertility

Chapter 2: Basics and Guidelines of the PCOS Diet — 13-16
- Balancing Macronutrients
- Managing Insulin Resistance
- Reducing Inflammation
- Importance of Fiber
- PCOS Superfoods

Chapter 3: Breakfast Delights — 17-22
- Energizing Smoothies and Shakes
- Protein-Packed Breakfast Bowls
- Overnight Oats and Chia Puddings
- Egg-cellent Breakfast Ideas

Chapter 4: Wholesome Lunches — 23-28
- Vibrant Salad Creations
- Nourishing Soups and Stews
- Satisfying Sandwiches and Wraps

Chapter 5: Dinners — 29-34
- Flavorful One-Pot Wonders
- Sheet Pan Suppers
- Stovetop Sensations

Chapter 6: Satisfying Snacks   35-38
- Crunchy and Crave-worthy
- Protein-Packed Power Bites
- Guilt-Free Treats

Chapter 7: Delectable Desserts   39-44
- Sweet Endings
- Decadent Delights
- Frozen Favorites

Chapter 8: PCOS-Friendly Beverages   45-52
- Hydration Station
- Herbal Infusions and Teas
- Smoothie and Juice Boosters

Chapter 9: Vegetarian and Vegan Entrées   53-66
- Plant-Powered Protein
- Flavorful Grain-Based Dishes
- Dairy-Free Delights

Chapter 10: Fish and Seafood Entrées   67-76
- Omega-3 Rich Recipes
- Quick and Easy Seafood Suppers
- Grilled and Baked Fish Favorites

Bonus: 30 days Meal Plan   77-84
Conclusion   85
Appendix   89-94

INTRODUCTION

In our fast-paced modern world, health often takes a backseat amidst the chaos of daily demands. Yet, within the challenges faced by millions of women lies a silent struggle, one that disrupts the delicate balance of hormones and wreaks havoc on their well-being. This struggle is Polycystic Ovary Syndrome (PCOS), a complex condition affecting up to 1 in 10 women worldwide.

PCOS isn't just a medical diagnosis; it's a silent adversary, manifesting in myriad symptoms that affect every aspect of a woman's life – from her physical health to her emotional well-being and even her dreams of motherhood. From the relentless battle with weight gain to the emotional rollercoaster of mood swings, from the frustration of irregular cycles to the heartache of infertility, PCOS casts a shadow over the lives of countless women, leaving them feeling lost, alone, and overwhelmed.

But amidst the darkness, there shines hope – the power of nutrition to heal, nourish, and restore balance from within. This is where "PCOS Diet Cookbook: The Complete Guide with Flavorful Recipes to Manage Polycystic Ovary Syndrome, Regulate your Hormones, and Improve Fertility" steps in.

This comprehensive guide is not just another cookbook; it's a lifeline for women facing the challenges of PCOS. With a deep understanding of the unique struggles faced by individuals with PCOS, this book offers more than just delicious recipes – it offers empowerment, support, and a pathway to reclaiming control over one's health and happiness.

Within these pages, you'll discover flavorful recipes meticulously crafted to support hormone balance, regulate insulin levels, and nourish your body from the inside out. From vibrant smoothie bowls bursting with antioxidants to comforting soups infused with healing herbs, each recipe shows the transformative power of food as medicine.

As you embark on this journey, let "PCOS Diet Cookbook" be your trusted companion, guiding you step by step towards a brighter, healthier future. Together, we'll journey towards better health and well-being, discovering the healing power of food for PCOS, one delicious recipe at a time.

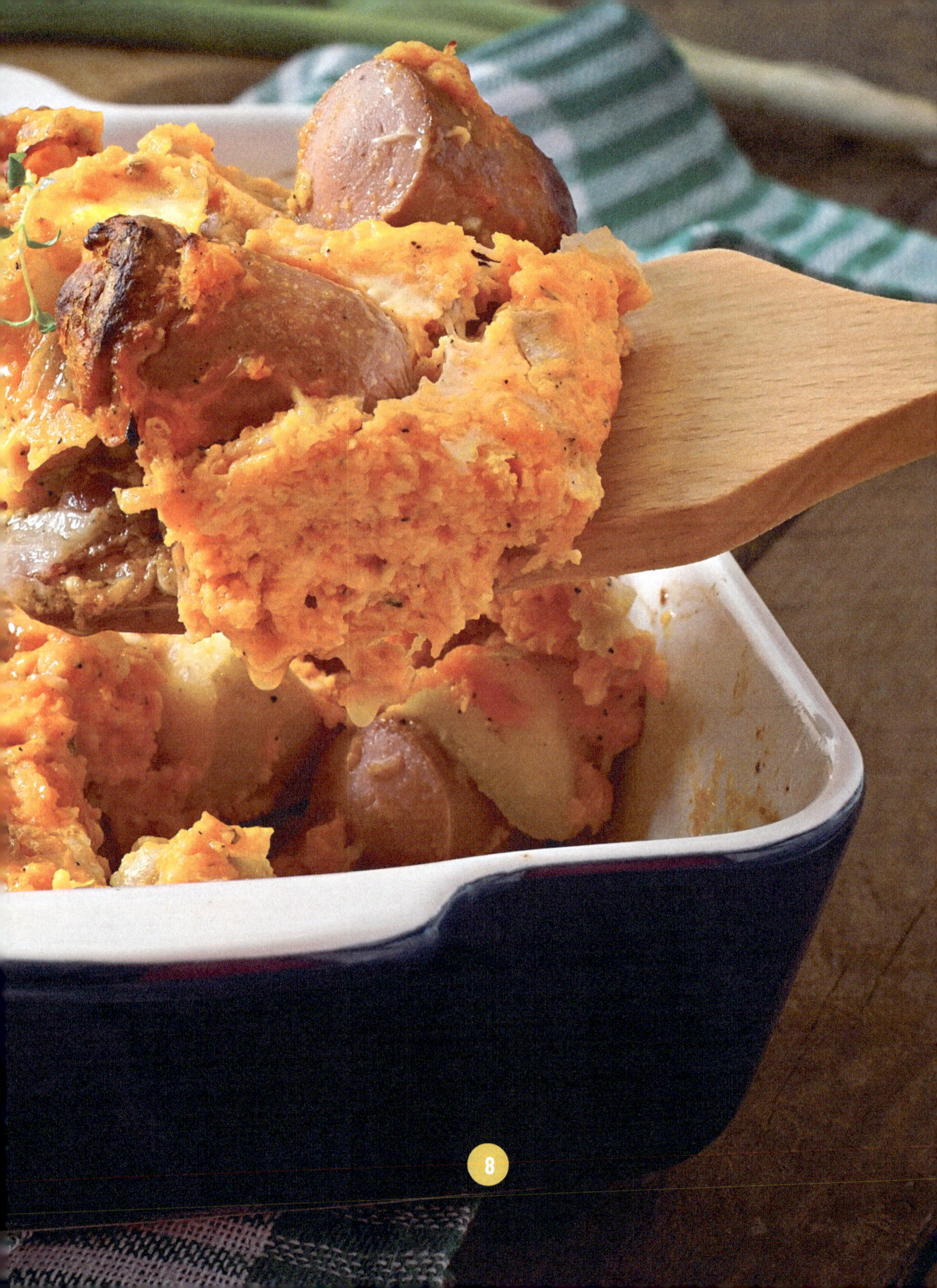

CHAPTER 1
DEMYSTIFYING PCOS

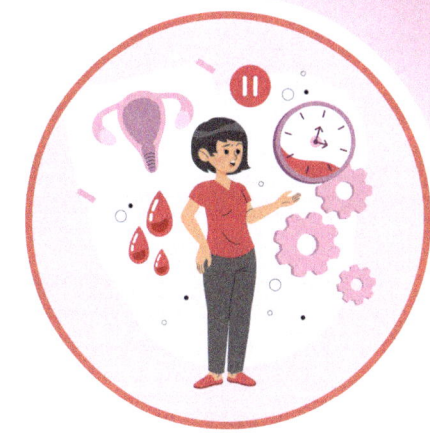

Alright, let's talk about PCOS - Polycystic Ovary Syndrome. It's more common than you might think.

PCOS isn't just about your ovaries - it's like a domino effect, affecting different parts of your body. Your metabolism, your skin, even your mood - they're all in on it. And while we don't have all the answers about what causes it, we do know that things like genetics, insulin resistance, and lifestyle factors can stir the pot.

So, if you've been dealing with irregular periods, stubborn weight gain, mood swings that rival a rollercoaster, or maybe trouble getting pregnant, you're not alone, sister. PCOS is like your body's way of saying, "Hey, I need a little extra attention over here!" But here's the thing: it's not your fault. PCOS is just one of those curveballs life throws our way. And the good news? There's plenty we can do to manage it and feel like our fabulous selves again.

What Causes PCOS?
PCOS, or Polycystic Ovary Syndrome, doesn't have a clear-cut cause, but it's thought to stem from a mix of genetic predisposition and environmental factors.

Here's a simplified breakdown:
Hormonal Imbalance: Women with PCOS typically have higher levels of male hormones, disrupting the normal ovulation process and leading to PCOS symptoms.
Insulin Resistance: Many women with PCOS also experience insulin resistance, where the body's cells don't respond effectively to insulin. This triggers the body to produce more insulin, which can further disrupt hormone levels and ovulation.
Genetics: PCOS often runs in families, suggesting a genetic link. If a close relative has PCOS, your risk may be higher.
Inflammation: Some studies suggest that chronic inflammation may contribute to PCOS development, aggravating insulin resistance and hormonal imbalances.
Lifestyle Factors: Unhealthy lifestyle choices like poor diet, lack of exercise, and being overweight can increase the likelihood of developing PCOS.

Symptoms and Diagnosis PCOS
Recognizing the signs of PCOS is crucial for getting the right help. Here's what to look out for:
i. Irregular Periods: PCOS often causes irregular menstrual cycles, with fewer than eight periods a year or unusually heavy or light bleeding.
ii. Weight Gain: PCOS can make it hard to shed extra pounds, especially around the abdomen, due to hormone imbalances like insulin resistance.
iii. Mood Swings: Fluctuating emotions, from highs to lows, are common with PCOS, making you feel like you're on an emotional rollercoaster.
iv. Unwanted Hair Growth: Excessive hair growth in unwanted places like the face or chest can be a symptom of PCOS, leaving you feeling self-conscious.
v. Acne: PCOS can lead to persistent acne breakouts, despite skincare efforts, affecting your confidence and skin health.
vi. Difficulty Getting Pregnant: If you're struggling to conceive, PCOS may be a factor due to its impact on ovulation.

Here's how doctors typically diagnose PCOS:

Symptom Check: If you're experiencing these symptoms, it's wise to discuss them with your doctor.
Medical History: Your doctor will ask about your menstrual history, weight changes, and other symptoms to assess the likelihood of PCOS.
Physical Exam: A pelvic exam may be conducted to check for signs like enlarged ovaries or unusual growths.
Blood Tests: These can reveal hormone levels, insulin resistance, and other markers associated with PCOS.
Ultrasound: An ultrasound of the pelvis can reveal cysts or other irregularities on the ovaries, aiding in diagnosis.

Treatment Options

Alright, let's talk about how we can tackle PCOS head-on and reclaim our health and happiness. There are a few different paths we can take, so let's explore our options:

1. Medical Interventions: Sometimes, a little extra help from the medical pros is just what we need.

Here are a few common treatments your doctor might recommend:
- **Birth Control Pills:** These can help regulate your menstrual cycle and reduce symptoms like acne and unwanted hair growth.
- **Metformin:** If you're dealing with insulin resistance, your doctor might prescribe metformin to help your body use insulin more effectively.
- **Fertility Treatments:** If you're trying to get pregnant, your doctor might recommend fertility medications or procedures to help you on your journey.

2. Lifestyle Modifications: Sometimes, small tweaks to our daily routine can make a world of difference.

Here are a few lifestyle changes to consider:
- **Exercise:** Getting moving can help improve insulin sensitivity and boost your mood. Whether it's yoga, walking, or dancing around your living room, find something you love and stick with it!
- **Stress Management:** Stress can wreak havoc on our hormones, so finding ways to unwind is key. Whether it's meditation, journaling, or curling up with a good book, make self-care a priority.
- **Sleep:** Getting enough shut-eye is crucial for hormone balance and overall well-being. Aim for 7-9 hours of quality sleep each night, and your body will thank you.

3. Dietary Strategies: Food - one of life's greatest pleasures!

Here are a few ways we can use nutrition to our advantage:
- **Balanced Meals:** Focus on filling your plate with a variety of nutrient-dense foods, like fruits, veggies, whole grains, lean proteins, and healthy fats. It's like giving your body a big hug from the inside out!
- **Fiber-Rich Foods:** Fiber is your friend! It helps keep your blood sugar stable and your digestion on track. Think fruits, veggies, legumes, and whole grains.
- **Hormone-Regulating Foods:** Certain foods can help support hormone balance and ease PCOS symptoms. Think leafy greens, fatty fish, nuts, seeds, and berries.

The Role of Diet in Managing PCOS

let's chat about how the food on your plate can play a big role in managing PCOS and helping you feel your best. Get ready to discover the power of nutrition!

Managing Insulin Resistance:
Conquering insulin resistance is a crucial step in managing PCOS symptoms. Let's look deeper into dietary strategies to enhance insulin sensitivity:

- **Low-Glycemic Goodness:** Opt for low-glycemic foods like non-starchy vegetables, whole grains, and legumes to stabilize blood sugar levels and curb insulin spikes.

- **Sugar Savvy:** Bid farewell to added sugars lurking in processed foods and sugary beverages. Instead, indulge in naturally sweet options like fruits to satisfy your sweet tooth while supporting stable blood sugar levels.

- **Pairing Power**: Combine carbohydrates with protein and fiber to slow down sugar absorption and promote steady energy levels throughout the day.

Reducing Inflammation:
Taming inflammation is key to easing PCOS symptoms. Let's explore dietary allies in the fight against inflammation:
- **Fatty Fish Feasts:** Incorporate omega-3-rich fish like salmon, mackerel, and sardines to quell inflammation and support overall health.

- **Green Goddesses:** Load up on leafy greens such as spinach, kale, and Swiss chard for their abundance of antioxidants and anti-inflammatory compounds.

- **Berry Bonanza:** Indulge in antioxidant-packed berries like blueberries, strawberries, and raspberries to combat inflammation and promote cellular health.

Hormone-Regulating Foods:
Harness the power of hormone-regulating foods to restore balance and harmony within your body. Here's a glimpse into nature's pharmacy:
- **Flaxseed Fix:** Incorporate flaxseeds into your diet for their rich lignan content, which supports estrogen regulation and hormonal equilibrium.
- **Minty Marvel:** Sip on spearmint tea to reduce excess androgens and alleviate symptoms like unwanted hair growth.
- **Cinnamon Charm:** Sprinkle cinnamon liberally in your meals to enhance insulin sensitivity and regulate menstrual cycles in women with PCOS.

Impact of PCOS on Fertility

Understanding how PCOS affects fertility is crucial for those navigating the journey towards conception.

Here's what you need to know:
- **Disrupted Ovulation:** One of the hallmark features of PCOS is irregular ovulation or anovulation, which can make it difficult to conceive. Without regular ovulation, the release of mature eggs necessary for fertilization becomes unpredictable, complicating conception efforts.

- **Hormonal Imbalance:** The hormonal imbalance characteristic of PCOS, including elevated levels of androgens (male hormones) and insulin resistance, further complicates fertility. These hormonal disruptions can interfere with the delicate hormonal dance necessary for ovulation and successful conception.

- **Irregular Menstrual Cycles:** Irregular menstrual cycles, a hallmark of PCOS, can hinder fertility by making it difficult to determine the most fertile times for conception. Without the predictability of a regular cycle, timing intercourse to coincide with ovulation becomes a challenge.

- **Increased Risk of Miscarriage:** Women with PCOS face an increased risk of miscarriage compared to women without the condition.

  The underlying hormonal imbalances and metabolic disturbances associated with PCOS can contribute to a higher risk of pregnancy complications, including miscarriage.

- **Challenges with Assisted Reproductive Technologies (ART):** While fertility treatments such as ovulation induction and in vitro fertilization (IVF) offer hope to women with PCOS struggling to conceive, they come with their own set of challenges.

  Women with PCOS may require higher doses of fertility medications and are at increased risk of ovarian hyperstimulation syndrome (OHSS) during ART procedures.

CHAPTER 2

BASICS AND GUIDELINES OF THE PCOS DIET

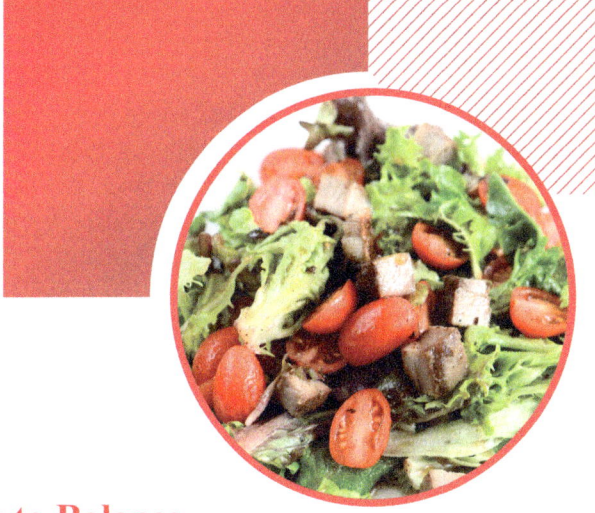

In this chapter, we'll look into the fundamental principles of the PCOS diet, equipping you with the knowledge and tools to nourish your body effectively.

Balancing Macronutrients

Understanding the significance of protein, healthy fats, and carbohydrates in your PCOS diet is key to promoting hormonal balance and managing symptoms effectively.

Importance of Protein, Healthy Fats, and Carbohydrates:
- **Protein Power:** Protein plays a crucial role in hormone synthesis, tissue repair, and satiety regulation. Incorporating lean sources of protein such as poultry, fish, tofu, and legumes into your meals can help stabilize blood sugar levels and promote feelings of fullness.

- **Healthy Fats:** Don't fear the fat! Healthy fats like avocados, nuts, seeds, and olive oil are essential for hormone production, brain function, and nutrient absorption. Including a variety of these fats in your diet can support hormone balance and overall health.

- **Carbohydrate Consciousness:** While carbohydrates often get a bad rap, they're an important source of energy and nutrients. Opt for complex carbohydrates like whole grains, fruits, vegetables, and legumes, which provide fiber and essential vitamins and minerals without causing rapid spikes in blood sugar.

How to Balance Macronutrients in PCOS Diet:

Achieving the right balance of macronutrients is crucial for managing PCOS symptoms effectively.

Here's how to strike that balance:
- **Protein Portioning:** Aim to include a palm-sized portion of protein in each meal and snack. This could include options like grilled chicken breast, salmon fillet, tofu scramble, or Greek yogurt.
- **Fat Focus:** Incorporate healthy fats into your meals by drizzling olive oil over salads, adding avocado slices to sandwiches, or sprinkling nuts and seeds onto yogurt or oatmeal.
- **Carb Consideration:** Fill your plate with plenty of non-starchy vegetables, leafy greens, and colorful fruits, and opt for whole grains like quinoa, brown rice, and oats. Be mindful of portion sizes and aim to include a variety of nutrient-dense carbohydrates in your diet.

Managing Insulin Resistance

In this section, we'll look into understanding insulin resistance in the context of PCOS and explore dietary strategies to enhance insulin sensitivity, promoting better metabolic health and symptom management.

What is Insulin Resistance?:
Insulin resistance, a cornerstone of PCOS, occurs when cells exhibit reduced responsiveness to insulin's regulatory signals.

This phenomenon disrupts glucose metabolism, leading to elevated blood sugar levels and metabolic dysfunction. In the context of PCOS, insulin resistance fuels hormonal imbalances, exacerbating symptoms like irregular menstrual cycles, weight gain, and fertility challenges.

Insulin's Role in PCOS:
Within the context of PCOS, insulin plays a multifaceted role, influencing hormonal dynamics and metabolic processes. Elevated insulin levels stimulate the ovaries to produce excess androgens, perpetuating hormonal imbalances and contributing to the manifestation of PCOS symptoms. Moreover, insulin resistance heightens the risk of metabolic comorbidities, underscoring the importance of targeted intervention.

Impact on Metabolic Health:
Beyond its immediate effects on reproductive health, insulin resistance poses a formidable risk to long-term metabolic well-being. Individuals with PCOS face an increased susceptibility to conditions such as type 2 diabetes, cardiovascular disease, and non-alcoholic fatty liver disease (NAFLD).

Dietary Strategies to Enhance Insulin Sensitivity

- **Embrace Low-Glycemic Foods:**

Opt for nutrient-dense, low-glycemic index (GI) foods to stabilize blood sugar levels and promote insulin sensitivity. Incorporate a colorful array of non-starchy vegetables, whole grains, legumes, and fruits with a lower sugar content into your daily meals.

- **Mindful Carbohydrate Consumption:**

Strike a delicate balance in carbohydrate consumption by distributing intake evenly throughout the day. Pair carbohydrates with lean proteins and healthy fats to mitigate blood sugar spikes and foster sustained energy release. Choose whole, unprocessed grains and prioritize complex carbohydrates over refined options.

- **Limit Sugary Temptations:**

Exercise prudence in navigating sugary temptations, steering clear of processed snacks, sugary beverages, and refined carbohydrates. These culprits can exacerbate insulin resistance and undermine metabolic health. Instead, indulge in naturally sweet options and savor the sweetness of whole fruits.

- **Harness the Power of Fiber:**

Elevate your dietary fiber intake with an abundance of plant-based foods, including vegetables, fruits, legumes, and whole grains. Fiber acts as a bulwark against blood sugar spikes, promoting satiety and aiding in digestive health. Prioritize fiber-rich options to support metabolic resilience.

- **Prioritize Protein and Healthy Fats:**

Elevate your meals with lean protein sources and healthy fats to enhance satiety and stabilize blood sugar levels. Incorporate lean meats, fatty fish, tofu, nuts, seeds, and olive oil into your culinary repertoire, crafting nourishing meals that support metabolic balance.

Reducing Inflammation

Inflammation, a hallmark of PCOS, fuels a cascade of physiological disturbances, exacerbating symptoms and undermining overall health.

Chronic inflammation not only perpetuates hormonal imbalances but also contributes to metabolic dysfunction and exacerbates symptoms like insulin resistance, weight gain, and fertility challenges. Hence, we need to ensure that we reduce inflammation.

Inflammatory Foods to Avoid:
To mitigate inflammation and its deleterious effects, it's crucial to steer clear of pro-inflammatory dietary culprits.

Here are some foods to minimize or avoid:
- **Processed Foods:** Refined carbohydrates, sugary snacks, and processed meats are notorious instigators of inflammation. Opt for whole, unprocessed foods whenever possible to reduce your intake of inflammatory additives and preservatives.
- **Trans Fats:** Say goodbye to trans fats found in fried foods, baked goods, and margarine. These artificial fats promote inflammation and pose a significant risk to metabolic health.
- **Sugary Treats:** Indulging in sweets like candies, pastries, and sugary drinks can cause inflammation and disrupt blood sugar levels. To promote better health, it's best to minimize your intake of these sugary delights.

Anti-Inflammatory Foods to Include Embrace Nature's Pharmacy:
Incorporate an abundance of anti-inflammatory foods into your daily diet to combat inflammation and promote wellness.

Some nutrient-rich options to prioritize are:
- **Fatty Fish:** Salmon, mackerel, and sardines are packed with omega-3 fatty acids, known for their powerful anti-inflammatory effects. Aim to incorporate fatty fish into your meals at least twice a week to harness their health benefits.
- **Leafy Greens:** Boost your diet with nutrient-packed leafy greens like spinach, kale, and Swiss chard. They are packed with antioxidants and phytonutrients that combat inflammation.
- **Colorful Berries:** get varieties of berries, including blueberries, strawberries, and raspberries. These gems help neutralize free radicals and reduce inflammation throughout the body.
- **Spice it Up:** Incorporate inflammation-fighting spices into your culinary creations to add flavor and health benefits. Turmeric, ginger, garlic, and cinnamon are renowned for their anti-inflammatory properties and can easily be incorporated into soups, stews, curries, and teas.

Benefits of Fiber for PCOS
1. Gut Health Support:
Fiber acts as a prebiotic, nourishing the beneficial bacteria in your gut and promoting a healthy microbiome. By fostering a thriving ecosystem of gut bacteria, fiber helps support digestion, nutrient absorption, and immune function, which are crucial aspects of managing PCOS symptoms.

2. Blood Sugar Regulation:
Soluble fiber slows down the absorption of glucose in the bloodstream, preventing rapid spikes in blood sugar levels and promoting stable energy levels throughout the day. By blunting the postprandial rise in blood sugar, fiber helps mitigate insulin resistance and supports glycemic control in individuals with PCOS.

3. Satiety Promotion:
High-fiber foods are inherently filling and satiating, helping you feel fuller for longer periods and reducing the likelihood of overeating or snacking on calorie-dense foods. By promoting satiety, fiber can aid in weight management efforts, which is particularly beneficial for individuals with PCOS who may struggle with excess weight.

4. Hormonal Balance:
Fiber plays a crucial role in estrogen metabolism, facilitating the elimination of excess hormones from the body. By promoting regular bowel movements and enhancing detoxification pathways, fiber helps maintain hormonal balance and may alleviate symptoms such as irregular menstrual cycles and hormonal fluctuations in individuals with PCOS.

High-Fiber Food Sources

1. Whole Grains:
Opt for whole grains such as oats, quinoa, brown rice, barley, and whole wheat, which are rich sources of dietary fiber. These grains provide a steady release of energy and are versatile ingredients that can be incorporated into a variety of savory and sweet dishes.

2. Legumes:
Beans, lentils, chickpeas, and peas are excellent sources of both soluble and insoluble fiber, as well as plant-based protein. Add legumes to soups, salads, stews, and curries to boost fiber intake and enhance nutritional value.

3. Fruits and Vegetables:
Load up on a colorful array of fruits and vegetables, which are naturally rich in fiber, vitamins, minerals, and antioxidants. Berries, apples, pears, broccoli, spinach, kale, and Brussels sprouts are particularly high-fiber choices that can be enjoyed in a variety of dishes.

4. Nuts and Seeds:
Incorporate nuts and seeds such as almonds, walnuts, chia seeds, flaxseeds, and pumpkin seeds into your diet as nutrient-dense sources of fiber, healthy fats, and essential micronutrients. Sprinkle them on salads, yogurt, oatmeal, or enjoy them as a satisfying snack.

List of Hormone-Regulating Foods

1. Flaxseeds:
- **Benefits:** Rich in lignans and omega-3 fatty acids, flaxseeds support estrogen metabolism and exert anti-inflammatory effects. They may help alleviate menstrual irregularities and promote hormonal balance in individuals with PCOS.

2. Spearmint:
- **Benefits:** Spearmint possesses anti-androgenic properties, which may help reduce excess testosterone levels in women with PCOS. Consuming spearmint tea or incorporating fresh spearmint leaves into your diet may help manage symptoms like hirsutism (unwanted hair growth).

3. Cinnamon:
- **Benefits:** Cinnamon is known for its insulin-sensitizing properties, making it beneficial for individuals with PCOS who struggle with insulin resistance. Incorporating cinnamon into your diet may help improve insulin sensitivity and regulate blood sugar levels.

4. Berries:
- **Benefits:** Berries such as blueberries, strawberries, and raspberries are rich in antioxidants, vitamins, and fiber. They help combat oxidative stress, reduce inflammation, and support overall health and well-being in individuals with PCOS.

5. Salmon:
- **Benefits:** Fatty fish like salmon are excellent sources of omega-3 fatty acids, which have anti-inflammatory properties and support hormone production and balance. Including salmon in your diet may help reduce inflammation and alleviate symptoms of PCOS.

6. Spinach:
- **Benefits:** Spinach is packed with nutrients like folate, iron, and vitamin K, which are essential for reproductive health and hormone regulation. Its antioxidant properties help combat oxidative stress, while its fiber content supports gut health and insulin sensitivity.

CHAPTER 3

BREAKFASTS

Welcome to a nourishing start to your day! These breakfast recipes are carefully crafted to support individuals managing PCOS, providing a balanced blend of nutrients to fuel your morning routine while promoting hormonal balance and stable blood sugar levels.

Berry Blast Smoothie

Servings: 2   Prep time: 5 min   Total time: 5 min

Nutrition per Serving: Calories: 150, Protein: 5g, Carbohydrates: 25g, Fat: 3g, Fiber: 6g

 **Ingredients**

 **Directions**

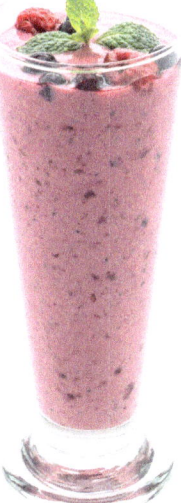

- 1 cup mixed berries (strawberries, blueberries, raspberries)
- 1/2 ripe banana
- 1/2 cup Greek yogurt
- 1 tablespoon flaxseeds
- 1 cup spinach leaves
- 1/2 cup almond milk
- Ice cubes (optional)

- Combine all ingredients in a blender.
- Blend until smooth and creamy.
- Pour into glasses and serve immediately.

Green Goddess Shake

Servings: 2   Prep time: 5 min   Total time: 5 min

Nutrition per Serving: Calories: 180, Protein: 6g, Carbohydrates: 15g, Fat: 12g, Fiber: 7g

 **Ingredients**

 Directions

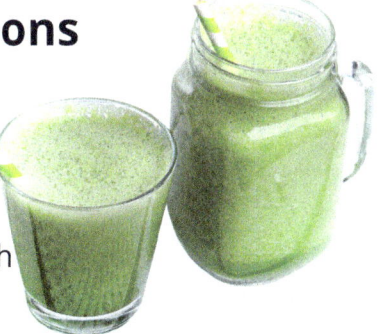

- 1 ripe avocado
- 1 cup spinach
- 1/2 cucumber, peeled and chopped
- 1/4 cup parsley leaves
- 1 tablespoon chia seeds
- 1 tablespoon honey (optional)
- 1 cup coconut water
- Ice cubes (optional)

- Combine all ingredients in a blender.
- Blend until smooth and velvety.
- Pour into glasses, garnish with a sprinkle of chia seeds, and serve.

Tropical Paradise Smoothie

Servings: 2   Prep time: 5 min   Total time: 5 min

Nutrition per Serving: Calories: 160, Protein: 3g, Carbohydrates: 20g, Fat: 9g, Fiber: 5g

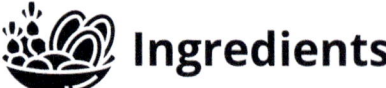 ### Ingredients

 ### Directions

- 1/2 cup pineapple chunks
- 1/2 cup mango chunks
- 1/2 ripe banana
- 1/2 cup coconut milk
- 1/4 cup Greek yogurt
- 1 tablespoon shredded coconut
- Ice cubes (optional)

- Blend all ingredients until smooth and creamy.
- Pour into glasses, garnish with a sprinkle of shredded coconut, and enjoy!

Peanut Butter Power Shake

Servings: 2   Prep time: 5 min   Total time: 5 min

Nutrition per Serving: Calories: 200, Protein: 8g, Carbohydrates: 15g, Fat: 14g, Fiber: 4g

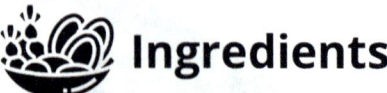 ### Ingredients

 ### Directions

- 1 ripe avocado
- 1 cup spinach
- 1/2 cucumber, peeled and chopped
- 1/4 cup parsley leaves
- 1 tablespoon chia seeds
- 1 tablespoon honey (optional)
- 1 cup coconut water
- Ice cubes (optional)

- Combine all ingredients in a blender.
- Blend until smooth and velvety.
- Pour into glasses, garnish with a sprinkle of chia seeds, and serve.

Vanilla Almond Overnight Oats

 Servings: 2	 Prep time: 5 min		 Total time: overnight

Nutrition per Serving: Calories: 300, Protein: 10g, Carbohydrates: 40g, Fat: 12g, Fiber: 8g

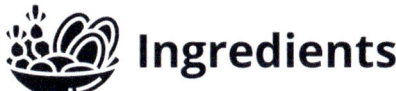 **Ingredients**

 **Directions**

- 1 cup rolled oats
- 1 cup unsweetened almond milk
- 1 tablespoon chia seeds
- 1 tablespoon almond butter
- 1 teaspoon vanilla extract
- 1/2 teaspoon cinnamon
- 1 tablespoon chopped almonds (for garnish)
- Fresh berries (optional, for topping)

- In a bowl or jar, combine rolled oats, almond milk, chia seeds, almond butter, vanilla extract, and cinnamon. Stir well to combine.
- Cover the bowl or jar and refrigerate overnight, or for at least 4 hours, to allow the oats to soften and the flavors to meld.
- Before serving, give the oats a good stir and adjust the consistency with additional almond milk if desired.
- Top with chopped almonds and fresh berries, if using, and enjoy this delightful and satisfying breakfast.

Tips for Adding Flavor Without Added Sugar:
Enhance the flavor of your overnight oats and chia puddings with these simple tips and tricks, allowing you to enjoy a delicious breakfast without relying on added sugar:

- **Natural Sweeteners:** Opt for natural sweeteners such as mashed banana, pureed dates, or a drizzle of honey or maple syrup to add sweetness without the need for refined sugar.
- **Flavor Extracts:** Experiment with flavor extracts like vanilla, almond, or coconut to infuse your breakfast with delicious aroma and taste, without any added sugar.
- **Spices and Herbs:** Sprinkle your overnight oats or chia puddings with warming spices like cinnamon, nutmeg, or ginger, or add fresh herbs like mint or basil for a burst of flavor and freshness.
- **Citrus Zest:** Grate some lemon or orange zest over your breakfast for a citrusy zing that brightens up the flavors and adds depth without the need for sugar.

Creamy Coconut Chia Pudding

 Servings: 2	 Prep time: 5 min		 Total time: overnight

Nutrition per Serving: Calories: 250, Protein: 6g, Carbohydrates: 20g, Fat: 15g, Fiber: 8g

Ingredients

- 1/4 cup chia seeds
- 1 cup unsweetened coconut milk
- 1 tablespoon unsweetened shredded coconut
- 1/2 teaspoon vanilla extract
- Pinch of sea salt
- Fresh fruit, for topping (optional)

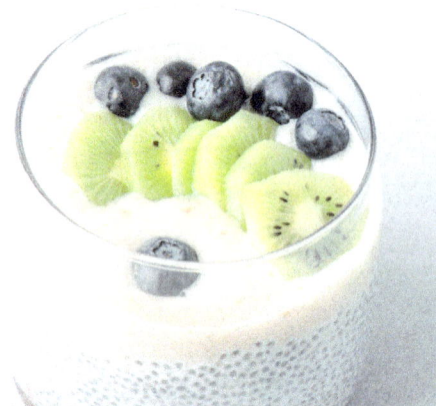

Directions

- In a bowl or jar, combine chia seeds, coconut milk, shredded coconut, vanilla extract, and a pinch of sea salt. Stir well to combine.
- Cover the bowl or jar and refrigerate overnight, allowing the chia seeds to absorb the liquid and form a pudding-like consistency.
- Before serving, give the chia pudding a good stir to evenly distribute the ingredients. If the pudding is too thick, add a splash of coconut milk to reach your desired consistency.
- Serve the chia pudding topped with fresh fruit or additional shredded coconut, if desired, and savor the creamy, coconutty goodness

Tips for Adding Flavor Without Added Sugar
Elevate the flavor of your overnight oats and chia puddings with these clever tips, ensuring a delicious breakfast experience without relying on added sugar::
- **Nut Butters:** Incorporate natural nut butters like almond butter or cashew butter into your recipes for added richness and creaminess, without the need for sugar.
- **Cocoa Powder:** Add a tablespoon of unsweetened cocoa powder to your overnight oats or chia puddings for a decadent chocolatey flavor, minus the added sugar.
- **Essence Extracts:** Enhance the flavor profile of your breakfasts with essence extracts such as almond, coconut, or orange, adding depth and complexity to your dishes without sugar.

Spinach and Feta Omelet

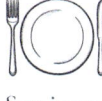 Servings: 1	 Prep time: 5 min	 Cook time: 5 min	 Total time: 10 min

Nutrition per Serving: Calories: 250, Protein: 20, Carbohydrates: 4g, Fat: 18g, Fiber: 2g

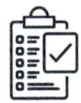 Ingredients

- 2 large eggs
- 1 cup fresh spinach leaves
- 1/4 cup crumbled feta cheese
- 1 tablespoon olive oil
- Salt and pepper, to taste
- Fresh herbs, for garnish (optional)

Suggestions for Boosting Nutrient Content:
- **Leafy Greens:** Amp up the nutrient density of your breakfast by adding leafy greens like kale, Swiss chard, or arugula to your egg scrambles, omelets, or frittatas for an extra dose of vitamins and antioxidants.
- **Lean Proteins:** Pair your eggs with lean proteins such as turkey sausage, smoked salmon, or grilled chicken breast to increase satiety and support muscle repair and growth.
- **Whole Grains:** Serve your egg dishes with a side of whole grains like quinoa, brown rice, or whole grain toast to add complex carbohydrates and fiber for sustained energy.

Directions

- In a bowl, whisk together the eggs until well beaten. Season with salt and pepper to taste.
- Apply heat to the olive oil in a non-stick skillet over medium heat. Add the spinach leaves and sauté until wilted, about 1-2 minutes.
- Pour the beaten eggs into the skillet, swirling to evenly distribute.
- Cook the omelet for 2-3 minutes, or until the edges start to set. Sprinkle the crumbled feta cheese evenly over the top.
- Using a spatula, fold the omelet in half and continue cooking for another 1-2 minutes, or until the cheese is melted and the eggs are cooked through.
- Slide the omelet onto a plate, garnish with fresh herbs if desired, and serve hot.

Veggie-Packed Breakfast Scramble

 Servings: 1	 Prep time: 10 min	 Cook time: 10 min	 Total time: 20 min

Nutrition per Serving: Calories: 280, Protein: 18, Carbohydrates: 10g, Fat: 20g, Fiber: 3g

Ingredients

- 4 large eggs
- 1 cup diced mixed vegetables (bell peppers, onions, mushrooms, spinach)
- 2 tablespoons grated cheese (cheddar, feta, or goat cheese)
- 1 tablespoon olive oil or butter
- Salt and pepper, to taste
- Fresh herbs, for garnish (optional)

Directions

- In a skillet, heat the olive oil or butter over medium heat. Add the diced vegetables and sauté until tender, about 5-7 minutes.
- In a bowl, whisk together the eggs until frothy. Season with salt and pepper to taste.
- Pour the beaten eggs into the skillet with the sautéed vegetables. Cook, stirring occasionally, until the eggs are softly set, about 3-4 minutes.
- Sprinkle the grated cheese over the top of the scramble and continue cooking for another 1-2 minutes, or until the cheese is melted and the eggs are cooked through.
- Transfer the scramble to serving plates, garnish with fresh herbs if desired, and serve hot.

Suggestions for Boosting Nutrient Content:

- **Omega-3 Boost:** Incorporate omega-3 rich ingredients such as flaxseeds, chia seeds, or fatty fish like salmon into your egg dishes to support hormone regulation and reduce inflammation associated with PCOS.
- Fiber-Filled Additions: Mix in fiber-rich foods like beans, lentils, or whole grains such as quinoa or brown rice to your egg dishes to promote digestive health, stabilize blood sugar levels, and enhance feelings of fullness.

CHAPTER 4 WHOLESOME LUNCHES

Hormone-Balancing Quinoa Power Bowl

 Servings: 2	 Prep time: 15 min	 Cook time: 10 min	 Total time: 25 min

Nutrition per Serving: Calories: 350, Protein: 18g, Carbohydrates: 45g, Fat: 12g, Fiber: 8g

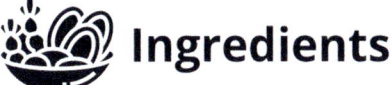 Ingredients

- 1 cup cooked quinoa
- 1 cup mixed greens (spinach, kale, arugula)
- 1/2 cup cooked chickpeas
- 1/2 avocado, sliced
- 1/4 cup shredded carrots
- 1/4 cup sliced cucumber
- 2 tablespoons pumpkin seeds
- 2 tablespoons crumbled feta cheese (optional)
- Lemon-tahini dressing (1 tablespoon tahini, 1 tablespoon lemon juice, 1 tablespoon water, salt, and pepper)

Directions

- In a large bowl, layer cooked quinoa, mixed greens, chickpeas, avocado slices, shredded carrots, sliced cucumber, pumpkin seeds, and crumbled feta cheese (if using).
- In a small bowl, whisk together the ingredients for the lemon-tahini dressing until smooth. Drizzle over the quinoa power bowl.
- Toss the ingredients gently to coat them with the dressing.
- Serve immediately and enjoy the nourishing flavors of this hormone-balancing quinoa power bowl.

Tips for Enhancement:

- **Hormone-Balancing Ingredients:** Enhance the bowl with hormone-balancing ingredients like leafy greens, chickpeas, avocado, and pumpkin seeds, which provide essential nutrients for PCOS management.
- **Lean Protein Addition:** Boost the protein content of the bowl by adding grilled chicken breast or tofu cubes for sustained energy and muscle support.
- **Variety and Flavor:** Experiment with different vegetables, herbs, and spices to add variety and depth of flavor to the power bowl. Consider adding roasted sweet potatoes, cherry tomatoes, or fresh herbs like cilantro or parsley for an extra burst of freshness.

Quinoa Salad with Citrus Dressing

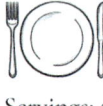 Servings: 2	 Prep time: 15 min	 Cook time: 10 min	 Total time: 25 min

Nutrition per Serving: Calories: 320, Protein: 12g, Carbohydrates: 40g, Fat: 14g, Fiber: 8g

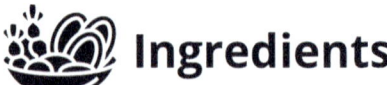 Ingredients

- 1 cup cooked quinoa
- 2 cups mixed greens (spinach, kale, arugula)
- 1/2 cup cooked edamame beans
- 1/2 cup shredded purple cabbage
- 1/4 cup sliced radishes
- 1/4 cup sliced almonds
- 1/2 orange, segmented
- 2 tablespoons crumbled goat cheese (optional)
- Citrus dressing (1 tablespoon olive oil, 1 tablespoon orange juice, 1 tablespoon lemon juice, 1 teaspoon honey, salt, and pepper)

Directions

- In a large bowl, combine cooked quinoa, mixed greens, edamame beans, shredded purple cabbage, sliced radishes, sliced almonds, and orange segments.
- In a small bowl, whisk together olive oil, orange juice, lemon juice, honey, salt, and pepper to create the citrus dressing.
- Drizzle the dressing over the salad ingredients and toss gently to coat.
- Sprinkle crumbled goat cheese (if using) over the salad.
- Serve immediately and enjoy the refreshing flavors and hormone-balancing goodness of this quinoa salad.

Tips for Enhancement:
- **Nutrient-Rich Additions:** Boost the nutritional value of the salad by adding hormone-balancing ingredients such as leafy greens, edamame beans, purple cabbage, and almonds.
- **Colorful Varieties:** Experiment with colorful vegetables and fruits to add variety and visual appeal to your salad. Try adding cherry tomatoes, bell peppers, or mandarin oranges for an extra pop of color and flavor.
- **Customizable Protein:** Customize your salad with your choice of protein, such as grilled chicken, shrimp, tofu, or chickpeas, to provide satiety and support muscle health.

Lentil and Sweet Potato Stew

 Servings: 4	 Prep time: 15 min	 Cook time: 40 min	 Total time: 55 min

Nutrition per Serving: Calories: 300, Protein: 15g, Carbohydrates: 45g, Fat: 8g, Fiber: 12g

Ingredients

- 1 tablespoon olive oil
- 1 onion, diced
- 2 cloves garlic, minced
- 2 carrots, diced
- 2 celery stalks, diced
- 1 large sweet potato, peeled and cubed
- 1 cup dried green lentils, rinsed
- 4 cups vegetable broth
- 1 can (14 oz) diced tomatoes
- 1 teaspoon ground turmeric
- 1 teaspoon ground cumin
- Salt and pepper, to taste
- Fresh parsley, for garnish

Directions

- In a large pot, heat olive oil over medium heat. Add diced onion, garlic, carrots, and celery, and cook until softened, about 5 minutes.
- Add cubed sweet potato, dried lentils, vegetable broth, diced tomatoes (with their juices), ground turmeric, and ground cumin. Season with salt and pepper to taste.
- Bring the stew to a boil, then reduce heat to low and simmer, covered, for 30-35 minutes or until lentils and sweet potatoes are tender.
- Once the stew is ready, adjust seasoning if needed and serve hot, garnished with fresh parsley.

Enhancements for PCOS Support:
- **Additional Hormone-Balancing Ingredients:** Incorporate ingredients like spinach or kale for added fiber and nutrients, as well as turmeric and cumin for their anti-inflammatory properties and hormone-balancing effects.
- **Lean Protein Addition:** Boost the protein content of the stew by adding diced chicken breast or tofu cubes, ensuring a well-rounded and satiating meal option.
- **Complex Carbohydrate Inclusions:** Add whole grains such as quinoa or barley to provide complex carbohydrates for sustained energy and blood sugar stability, complementing the hearty nature of the stew.
- **Incorporating Healthy Fats:** Drizzle each serving with a tablespoon of extra virgin olive oil or top with avocado slices to enhance the flavor and promote satiety through healthy fats.

Lentil and Spinach Soup

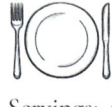 Servings: 4	 Prep time: 10 min	 Cook time: 35 min	 Total time: 50 min

Nutrition per Serving: Calories: 280, Protein: 14g, Carbohydrates: 45g, Fat: 6g, Fiber: 10g

Ingredients

- 1 tablespoon olive oil
- 1 onion, diced
- 2 cloves garlic, minced
- 2 carrots, diced
- 2 celery stalks, diced
- 1 cup dried green lentils, rinsed
- 4 cups vegetable broth
- 1 can (14 oz) diced tomatoes
- 2 cups chopped spinach
- 1 teaspoon ground cumin
- 1 teaspoon paprika
- Salt and pepper, to taste
- Fresh cilantro, for garnish

Directions

- Heat olive oil in a large pot over medium heat. Add diced onion, garlic, carrots, and celery, and sauté until softened, about 5 minutes.
- Add dried lentils, vegetable broth, diced tomatoes (with their juices), ground cumin, and paprika. Season with salt and pepper.
- Bring the soup to a boil, then reduce heat to low and simmer, covered, for 25-30 minutes or until lentils are tender.
- Stir in chopped spinach and continue to simmer for an additional 5 minutes until wilted.
- Adjust seasoning if needed and serve hot, garnished with fresh cilantro.

Enhancements for PCOS Support:
- **Additional Hormone-Balancing Ingredients:** Boost the soup's hormone-balancing properties by adding ground turmeric or ginger for anti-inflammatory benefits, as well as incorporating cruciferous vegetables like cauliflower or broccoli for their detoxifying properties.
- **Lean Protein Addition:** Enhance the protein content by adding cooked chicken breast or tofu cubes to provide sustained energy and support muscle health.
- **Complex Carbohydrate Inclusions:** Introduce complex carbohydrates such as barley or quinoa to promote stable blood sugar levels and increase satiety, complementing the soup's hearty texture.
- **Incorporating Healthy Fats:** Finish each serving with a drizzle of flaxseed oil or a sprinkle of hemp seeds to add essential omega-3 fatty acids and promote hormone balance.

Chickpea and Avocado Wrap

 Servings: 2	 Prep time: 15 min		 Total time: 15 min

Nutrition per Serving: Calories: 320, Protein: 12g, Carbohydrates: 40g, Fat: 14g, Fiber: 8g

Ingredients

- 1 can (15 oz) chickpeas, drained and rinsed
- 1 ripe avocado, mashed
- 1/4 cup diced cucumber
- 1/4 cup diced tomatoes
- 2 tablespoons diced red onion
- 2 tablespoons chopped fresh parsley
- Juice of 1/2 lemon
- Salt and pepper, to taste
- 2 whole grain or gluten-free wraps
- Handful of mixed greens

Directions

- In a mixing bowl, combine the mashed avocado, diced cucumber, tomatoes, red onion, chopped parsley, and lemon juice. Mix well to combine.
- Add the drained and rinsed chickpeas to the bowl and gently mash them with a fork, leaving some texture.
- Season the chickpea and avocado mixture with salt and pepper to taste.
- Lay out the wraps on a flat surface. Divide the chickpea and avocado mixture evenly between the wraps, spreading it out into a line down the center of each wrap.
- Top each wrap with a handful of mixed greens.
- Roll up the wraps tightly, folding in the sides as you go.
- Slice the wraps in half diagonally and serve immediately.

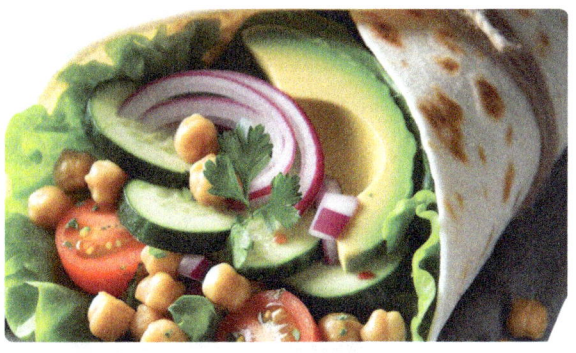

Enhancements for PCOS Support:
- **Incorporate Leafy Greens:** Boost the nutrient content and hormone-balancing properties of the wrap by adding a generous handful of leafy greens such as spinach or kale to each wrap.
- **Add Lean Protein:** Include a source of lean protein such as grilled chicken breast strips or tofu cubes to increase the protein content and create a more satisfying meal option.
- **Include Healthy Fats:** Enhance the satiety and hormone-balancing effects of the wrap by drizzling each serving with a tablespoon of extra virgin olive oil or sprinkling with hemp seeds for an added omega-3 boost.

Turkey and Hummus Wrap

 Servings: 2	 Prep time: 10 min		 Total time: 10 min

Nutrition per Serving: Calories: 320, Protein: 20g, Carbohydrates: 30g, Fat: 15g, Fiber: 5g

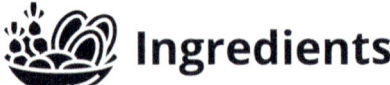 Ingredients

- 4 slices of roasted turkey breast
- 2 whole grain or gluten-free wraps
- 1/4 cup hummus
- 1/2 cucumber, thinly sliced
- 1/2 red bell pepper, thinly sliced
- Handful of baby spinach leaves

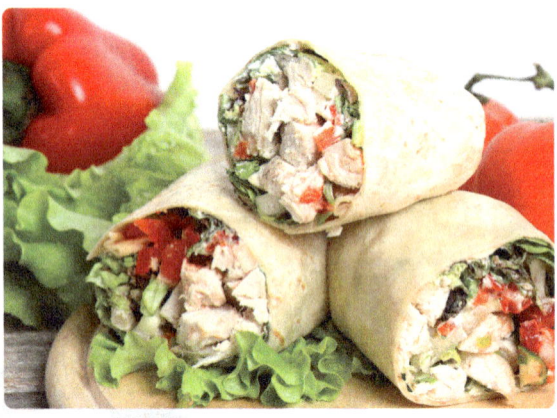

Directions

- Lay out the wraps on a flat surface. Spread a layer of hummus evenly over each wrap.
- Place two slices of roasted turkey breast on each wrap, covering the hummus layer.
- Arrange cucumber slices and red bell pepper strips on top of the turkey slices.
- Top each wrap with a handful of baby spinach leaves.
- Roll up the wraps tightly, folding in the sides as you go.
- Slice the wraps in half diagonally and serve immediately.

Enhancements for PCOS Support:
- **Include Leafy Greens:** Boost the nutrient content and hormone-balancing properties of the wrap by adding a generous handful of leafy greens such as arugula or kale to each wrap.
- **Add Healthy Fats:** Enhance the satiety and hormone-balancing effects of the wrap by adding sliced avocado or a sprinkle of hemp seeds for an added dose of omega-3 fatty acids.
- **Incorporate Colorful Vegetables:** Increase the antioxidant content and visual appeal of the wrap by adding vibrant vegetables such as shredded carrots or thinly sliced radishes for added crunch and flavor.
- **Experiment with Seasonings:** Explore different flavor profiles by adding a dash of ground cumin or smoked paprika to the hummus spread for a hint of warmth and depth.

CHAPTER 5

DINNERS

Wholesome One-Pot Quinoa Primavera

 Servings: 4    Prep time: 10 min   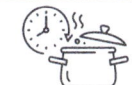 Cook time: 25 min    Total time: 35 min

Nutrition per Serving: Calories: 320, Protein: 12g, Carbohydrates: 50g, Fat: 8g, Fiber: 10g

Ingredients

- 1 tablespoon olive oil
- 1 onion, diced
- 2 cloves garlic, minced
- 2 carrots, diced
- 1 bell pepper, diced
- 1 zucchini, diced
- 1 cup quinoa, rinsed
- 2 cups vegetable broth
- 1 can (14 oz) diced tomatoes
- 1 teaspoon Italian seasoning
- Salt and pepper, to taste
- Fresh basil leaves, for garnish

Tips for Enhancement:
- **Include Healthy Fats:** Drizzle each serving with a tablespoon of extra virgin olive oil or sprinkle with chopped nuts or seeds for an added dose of healthy fats.
- **Experiment with Vegetables:** Customize the dish by incorporating your favorite seasonal vegetables or using frozen mixed vegetables for added convenience.

Directions

- In a large pot or skillet, heat olive oil over medium heat. Add diced onion and garlic, and cook until fragrant, about 2 minutes.
- Add diced carrots, bell pepper, and zucchini to the pot. Cook for another 5 minutes, stirring occasionally.
- Add rinsed quinoa to the pot and toast for 2 minutes, stirring frequently.
- Pour in vegetable broth and diced tomatoes (with their juices). Stir in Italian seasoning, salt, and pepper.
- Bring the mixture to a boil, then reduce heat to low. Cover and simmer for 15-20 minutes, or until quinoa is cooked and vegetables are tender.
- Remove from heat and let the quinoa primavera sit for a few minutes to allow flavors to meld.
- Serve hot, garnished with fresh basil leaves.

Hearty Lentil and Vegetable Stew

 Servings: 4	 Prep time: 10 min	 Cook time: 30 min	 Total time: 40 min

Nutrition per Serving: Calories: 320, Protein: 20g, Carbohydrates: 30g, Fat: 15g, Fiber: 5g

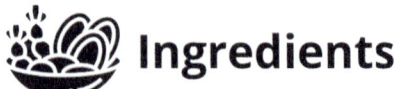 Ingredients

- 1 tablespoon olive oil
- 1 onion, diced
- 2 cloves garlic, minced
- 2 carrots, sliced
- 2 celery stalks, sliced
- 1 bell pepper, diced
- 1 cup dried green lentils, rinsed
- 4 cups vegetable broth
- 1 can (14 oz) diced tomatoes
- 1 teaspoon dried thyme
- Salt and pepper, to taste
- Fresh parsley, for garnish

Enhancements for PCOS Support:
- **Incorporate Leafy Greens:** Add a handful of chopped spinach or kale to the stew during the last few minutes of cooking for an extra boost of fiber, vitamins, and minerals.
- **Boost Protein Content:** Stir in cooked quinoa or diced tofu to increase the protein content and make the stew more filling and satisfying.
- **Experiment with Herbs:** Customize the flavor profile by adding fresh herbs like rosemary or basil for a fragrant and aromatic touch.
- **Include Healthy Fats:** Drizzle each serving with a teaspoon of flaxseed oil or sprinkle with hemp seeds for added omega-3 fatty acids and hormone-balancing benefits.

Directions

- In a large pot, heat olive oil over medium heat. Add diced onion and garlic, and sauté until softened, about 5 minutes.
- Add sliced carrots, celery, and diced bell pepper to the pot, and cook for an additional 5 minutes, stirring occasionally.
- Stir in rinsed lentils, vegetable broth, diced tomatoes (with their juices), dried thyme, salt, and pepper.
- Bring the stew to a boil, then reduce heat to low. Cover and simmer for 20-25 minutes, or until lentils and vegetables are tender.
- Adjust seasoning if needed. Serve hot, garnished with fresh parsley.

Lemon Herb Salmon and Vegetable Medley

 Servings: 4	 Prep time: 10 min	 Cook time: 20 min	 Total time: 30 min

<u>Nutrition per Serving:</u> Calories: 320, Protein: 25g, Carbohydrates: 20g, Fat: 15g, Fiber: 8g

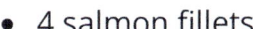 Ingredients

- 4 salmon fillets
- 2 cups broccoli florets
- 1 red bell pepper, sliced
- 1 yellow bell pepper, sliced
- 1 small zucchini, sliced
- 1 tablespoon olive oil
- 2 cloves garlic, minced
- 1 tablespoon fresh lemon juice
- 1 teaspoon lemon zest
- 1 teaspoon dried thyme
- Salt and pepper, to taste
- Fresh parsley, for garnish

Enhancements for PCOS Support:
- **Lean Protein:** Opt for wild-caught salmon fillets as a rich source of omega-3 fatty acids, essential for hormone balance and inflammation reduction.
- **Non-Starchy Vegetables:** Include colorful non-starchy vegetables like broccoli, bell peppers, and zucchini for fiber, vitamins, and antioxidants without causing blood sugar spikes.
- **Healthy Fats:** Enhance the meal's satiety and nutritional value with heart-healthy fats from olive oil and omega-3s from salmon.

Directions

- Preheat your oven to 400°F (200°C) and line a baking sheet with parchment paper.
- Arrange the salmon fillets in the center of the baking sheet and surround them with broccoli florets, bell pepper slices, and zucchini slices.
- In a small bowl, whisk together olive oil, minced garlic, lemon juice, lemon zest, dried thyme, salt, and pepper.
- Drizzle the lemon herb mixture over the salmon and vegetables, ensuring even coating.
- Roast in the preheated oven for 15-20 minutes, or until the salmon is cooked through and the vegetables are tender.
- Remove from the oven and garnish with fresh parsley before serving.

- **Balanced Seasonings:** Utilize fresh herbs, garlic, and citrus zest for flavor without relying on excess salt or added sugars, supporting overall health and wellness.

Vibrant Mediterranean Chicken and Veggie Delight

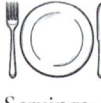 Servings: 4	 Prep time: 15 min	 Cook time: 25 min	 Total time: 40 min

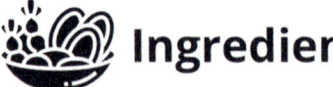 Ingredients

- 4 boneless, skinless chicken breasts
- 2 cups cherry tomatoes
- 1 red onion, sliced
- 1 yellow bell pepper, sliced
- 1 small eggplant, diced
- 1 tablespoon olive oil
- 2 cloves garlic, minced
- 1 tablespoon balsamic vinegar
- 1 teaspoon dried oregano
- Salt and pepper, to taste
- Fresh basil, for garnish

Nutrition per Serving:

Calories: 300, Protein: 28g, Carbohydrates: 20g, Fat: 12g, Fiber: 6g

Directions

- Preheat your oven to 400°F (200°C) and line a baking sheet with parchment paper.
- Place the chicken breasts in the center of the baking sheet and surround them with cherry tomatoes, sliced red onion, bell pepper slices, and diced eggplant.
- In a small bowl, whisk together olive oil, minced garlic, balsamic vinegar, dried oregano, salt, and pepper.
- Drizzle the olive oil mixture over the chicken and vegetables, ensuring even coating.
- Roast in the preheated oven for 20-25 minutes, or until the chicken is cooked through and the vegetables are tender.
- Remove from the oven and garnish with fresh basil before serving.

Enhancements for PCOS Support:
- **Colorful Vegetable Variety:** Incorporate a rainbow of vegetables like cherry tomatoes, bell peppers, red onions, and eggplant, rich in antioxidants, vitamins, and minerals.
- **Healthy Fat Addition:** Enhance the meal's flavor and satiety with heart-healthy monounsaturated fats from olive oil, contributing to hormone balance and overall well-being.
- **Herb and Vinegar Seasoning:** Utilize aromatic herbs like oregano and the tangy acidity of balsamic vinegar for flavorful seasoning without relying on excess salt or sugar.

Savory Shrimp Stir-Fry

 Servings: 4	 Prep time: 15 min	 Cook time: 10 min	 Total time: 25 min

<u>Nutrition per Serving:</u> Calories: 250, Protein: 20g, Carbohydrates: 15g, Fat: 10g, Fiber: 4g

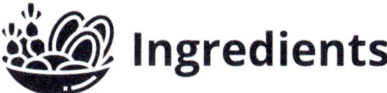 Ingredients

- 1 lb large shrimp, peeled and deveined
- 2 cups mixed vegetables (such as bell peppers, broccoli, snap peas)
- 2 cloves garlic, minced
- 1 tablespoon grated ginger
- 2 tablespoons low-sodium soy sauce
- 1 tablespoon sesame oil
- 1 teaspoon honey or maple syrup
- 1 tablespoon rice vinegar
- 2 green onions, thinly sliced
- Cooked brown rice or quinoa, for serving

Seasoning Suggestions:
- **Fresh Herbs and Spices:** Incorporate fresh herbs like cilantro or basil, along with spices such as red pepper flakes or ground black pepper, to add depth of flavor without excess sodium.
- **Citrus Zest:** Enhance the dish with a burst of freshness by adding lemon or lime zest, which adds bright citrusy notes without the need for additional salt.
- **Aromatics:** Use aromatic ingredients like garlic and ginger generously to infuse the stir-fry with irresistible fragrance and flavor.

 Directions

- In a small bowl, whisk together the minced garlic, grated ginger, low-sodium soy sauce, sesame oil, honey or maple syrup, and rice vinegar to make the sauce. Set aside.
- Heat a large skillet or wok over medium-high heat. Add a drizzle of oil and sauté the mixed vegetables until they are crisp-tender, about 3-4 minutes. Remove the vegetables from the skillet and set aside.
- In the same skillet, add the shrimp and cook until they turn pink and opaque, about 2-3 minutes per side.
- Return the cooked vegetables to the skillet with the shrimp. Pour the sauce over the shrimp and vegetables, tossing to coat evenly. Cook for an additional 1-2 minutes, until everything is heated through.
- Remove from heat and garnish with thinly sliced green onions. Serve the shrimp stir-fry hot over cooked brown rice or quinoa.

Flavorful Tofu and Vegetable Stir-Fry

 Servings: 4	 Prep time: 15 min	 Cook time: 15 min	 Total time: 30 min

Nutrition per Serving: Calories: 220, Protein: 15g, Carbohydrates: 20g, Fat: 10g, Fiber: 6g

Ingredients

- 1 block (14 oz) firm tofu, drained and cubed
- 2 cups mixed vegetables (such as bell peppers, broccoli, carrots, snow peas)
- 2 cloves garlic, minced
- 1 tablespoon grated ginger
- 2 tablespoons low-sodium soy sauce or tamari
- 1 tablespoon rice vinegar
- 1 tablespoon hoisin sauce
- 1 tablespoon sesame oil
- 2 green onions, thinly sliced
- Cooked brown rice or quinoa, for serving

Seasoning Suggestions:
- **Herbs and Spices:** Elevate the flavor profile with a combination of dried herbs like basil, oregano, and red pepper flakes, adding complexity without relying on salt.
- **Citrus Zest:** Brighten up the dish by incorporating citrus zest, such as lemon or orange, for a burst of freshness and aroma.
- **Umami Boosters:** Enhance the savory taste with umami-rich ingredients like mushrooms or nutritional yeast, providing depth and richness to the stir-fry.

Directions

- Heat a large skillet or wok over medium heat. Add the cubed tofu and cook until golden brown on all sides, about 5-7 minutes. Remove the tofu from the skillet and set aside.
- In the same skillet, add a drizzle of oil if needed and sauté the mixed vegetables until they are crisp-tender, about 3-4 minutes.
- Push the vegetables to one side of the skillet and add the minced garlic and grated ginger to the empty space. Cook for 30 seconds, until fragrant.
- Return the cooked tofu to the skillet with the vegetables.
- In a small bowl, whisk together the low-sodium soy sauce or tamari, rice vinegar, hoisin sauce, and sesame oil. Pour the sauce over the tofu and vegetables, tossing to coat evenly. Cook for an additional 2-3 minutes, until everything is heated through.
- Remove from heat and garnish with thinly sliced green onions. Serve the tofu and vegetable stir-fry hot over cooked brown rice or quinoa.

CHAPTER 6   SATISFYING SNACKS

Wholesome Trail Mix

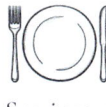 Servings: 4	 Prep time: 5 min	Portion Size: ¼ cup	 Total time: 5 min

<u>Nutrition per Serving</u>: Calories: 150, Protein: 5g, Carbohydrates: 12g, Fat: 10g, Fiber: 3g

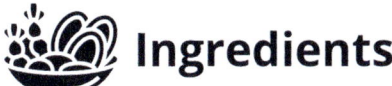 Ingredients

- 1 cup mixed nuts (almonds, walnuts, cashews)
- ½ cup dried fruit (raisins, cranberries, apricots)
- ¼ cup pumpkin seeds
- ¼ cup dark chocolate chips (optional)

Directions

- In a large bowl, combine mixed nuts, dried fruit, pumpkin seeds, and dark chocolate chips, if using.
- Toss the ingredients together until evenly distributed.
- Divide the trail mix into individual ¼ cup portions and store in small airtight containers for convenient snacking.

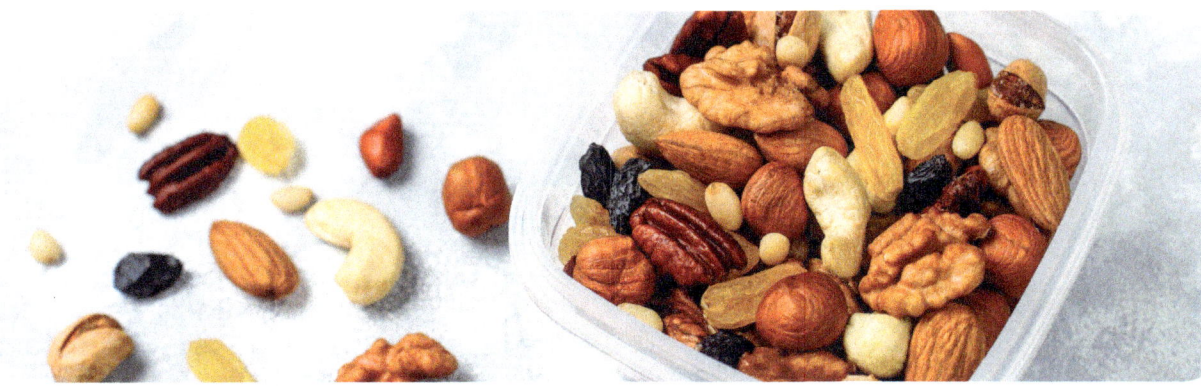

Portion Control Tips:
- **Pre-Portioned Packs:** Divide the trail mix into single-serving portions ahead of time to prevent overeating.
- **Use Small Bowls:** When serving, opt for smaller bowls or containers to visually control portion sizes.
- **Mindful Eating:** Take your time to enjoy each bite and savor the flavors, focusing on the sensory experience of eating.

Veggie and Hummus Snack Packs

 Servings: 4	 Prep time: 10 min	Portion Size: 1 cup vegetables + 2 tablespoons hummus	 Total time: 10 min

Nutrition per Serving: Calories: 120, Protein: 4g, Carbohydrates: 10g, Fat: 7g, Fiber: 4g

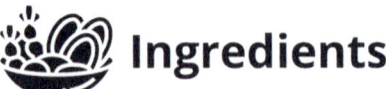 Ingredients

- 2 cups mixed vegetables (carrot sticks, cucumber slices, bell pepper strips, cherry tomatoes)
- ½ cup hummus (store-bought or homemade)

Directions

- Wash and prepare the mixed vegetables by cutting them into sticks, slices, or strips.
- Divide the mixed vegetables into individual snack-size containers or zip-top bags.
- Spoon 2 tablespoons of hummus into separate small containers or portion cups.
- Seal the containers tightly and store in the refrigerator until ready to enjoy.

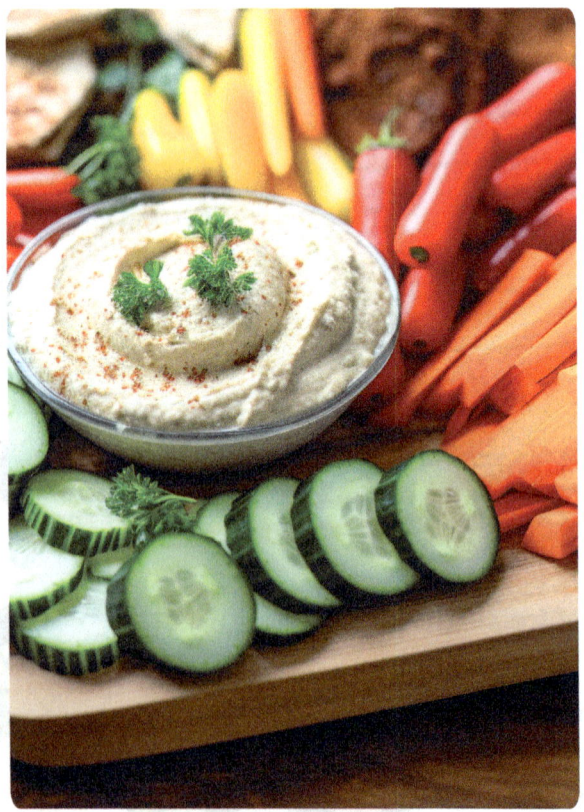

Portion Control Tips:
- **Pre-Portioned Containers:** Pack the vegetables and hummus into separate containers to ensure controlled portion sizes.
- **Visual Cues:** Aim for a colorful assortment of vegetables to make your snack visually appealing and satisfying.
- **Enjoy Mindfully:** Take the time to savor each bite, focusing on the flavors and textures of the vegetables and hummus.

Guilt-Free Sweet Treats

Berry Yogurt Parfait

Servings: 1   Prep time: 5 min   Total time: 5 min

Nutrition per Serving: Calories: 200, Protein: 15g, Carbohydrates: 25g, Fat: 5g, Fiber: 5g

Ingredients

- 1 cup Greek yogurt (plain, unsweetened)
- 1/2 cup mixed berries (strawberries, blueberries, raspberries)
- 1 tablespoon chopped nuts (almonds, walnuts)
- 1 teaspoon honey (optional)

Directions

- In a glass, layer Greek yogurt, mixed berries, and chopped nuts.
- Drizzle with honey if desired.
- Repeat the layers.
- Serve immediately or refrigerate for a refreshing dessert.

Dark Chocolate Almond Clusters

Servings: 8 clusters   Prep time: 10 min   Total time: 30 min

Nutrition per Serving: Calories: 120, Protein: 3g, Carbohydrates: 10g, Fat: 8g, Fiber: 2g

Ingredients

- 1/2 cup dark chocolate chips (70% cocoa or higher)
- 1/4 cup almonds, chopped
- Sea salt (optional)

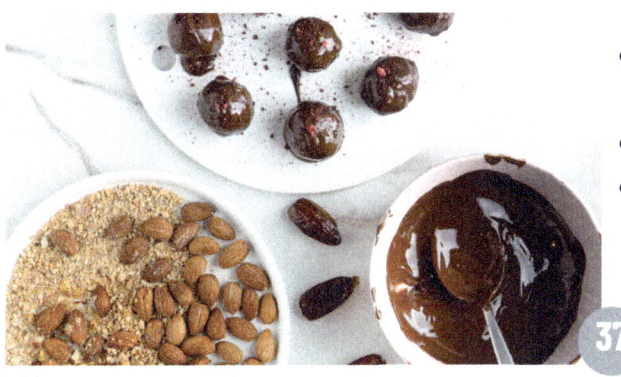

Directions

- Melt dark chocolate chips in a microwave-safe bowl in 30-second intervals, stirring until smooth.
- Stir in chopped almonds until well coated.
- Drop spoonfuls of the mixture onto a parchment-lined baking sheet.
- Sprinkle with sea salt if desired.
- Allow to cool and harden at room temperature or refrigerate for faster setting.
- Enjoy as a satisfying chocolatey treat!

Guilt-Free Savory Delights

Baked Sweet Potato Chips

Servings: 2   Prep time: 10 min   Total time: 30 min

Nutrition per Serving: Calories: 150, Protein: 2g, Carbohydrates: 25g, Fat: 5g, Fiber: 4g

Ingredients

- 1 large sweet potato, thinly sliced
- 1 tablespoon olive oil
- Sea salt to taste
- Optional: garlic powder, paprika, or other seasonings

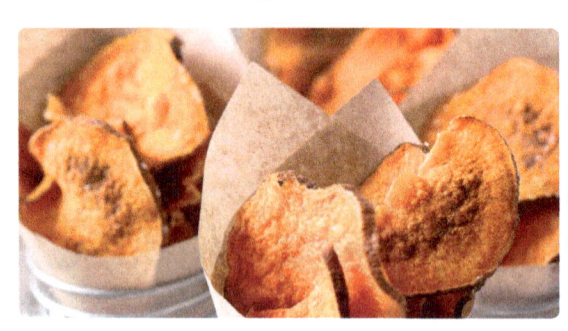

Directions

- Preheat oven to 375°F (190°C).
- Toss sweet potato slices with olive oil and seasonings in a bowl until evenly coated.
- Arrange slices in a single layer on a baking sheet lined with parchment paper.
- Bake for 15-20 minutes or until crispy, flipping halfway through.
- Sprinkle with sea salt while still warm.
- Allow to cool slightly before serving as a crunchy, guilt-free snack.

Veggie Stuffed Avocado

Servings: 2   Prep time: 10 min   Total time: 10 min

Nutrition per Serving: Calories: 200, Protein: 5g, Carbohydrates: 12g, Fat: 15g, Fiber: 7g

Ingredients

- 1 ripe avocado, halved and pitted
- 1/2 cup cherry tomatoes, halved
- 1/4 cup cucumber, diced
- 2 tablespoons feta cheese, crumbled (optional)
- Fresh basil leaves, chopped
- Balsamic glaze for drizzling

Directions

- Scoop out some of the avocado flesh to create a larger cavity.
- In a bowl, combine cherry tomatoes, cucumber, feta cheese, and basil.
- Spoon the veggie mixture into the avocado halves.
- Drizzle with balsamic glaze just before serving and Enjoy!

CHAPTER 7 — DELECTABLE DESSERTS

Lemon-Kissed Cinnamon Baked Apples

Servings: 4	Prep time: 10 min		Total time: 40 min

Nutrition per Serving: Calories: 120, Protein: 1g, Carbohydrates: 30g, Fat: 0.5g, Fiber: 5g

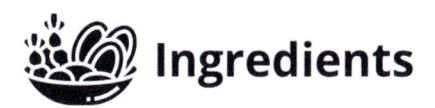

Ingredients

- 4 apples (such as Granny Smith or Honeycrisp)
- 2 tablespoons honey or maple syrup
- 1 teaspoon cinnamon
- 1 tablespoon lemon juice
- 1/4 teaspoon nutmeg
- 1/4 cup chopped walnuts or almonds (optional)
- Greek yogurt or coconut yogurt for serving

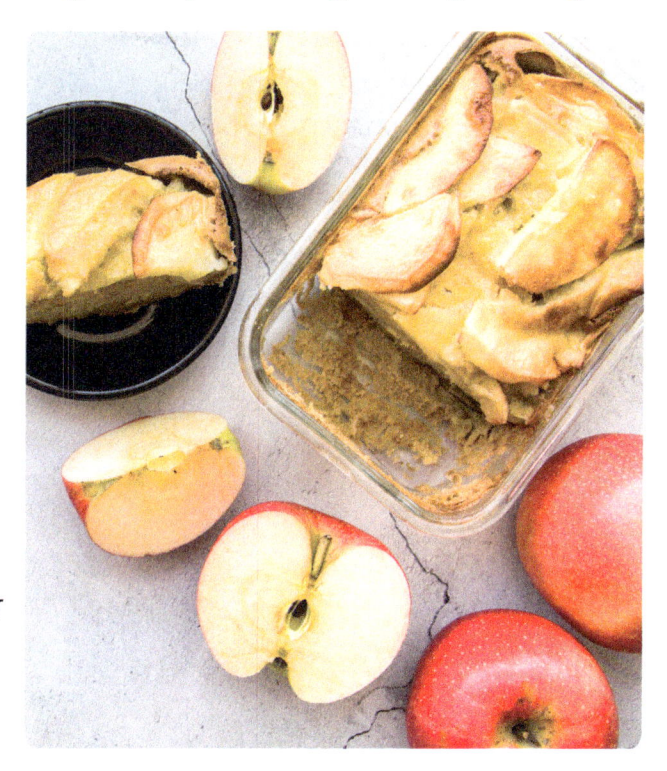

Directions

- Preheat your oven to 375°F (190°C).
- Core the apples and place them in a baking dish.
- In a small bowl, mix together the honey or maple syrup, cinnamon, lemon juice, and nutmeg.
- Spoon the mixture evenly into the centers of the apples.
- If using, sprinkle the chopped nuts over the top of each apple.
- Cover the baking dish with foil and bake for 30-35 minutes, or until the apples are tender.
- Serve warm with a dollop of Greek yogurt or coconut yogurt on top.

Veggie and Hummus Snack Packs

| Servings: 4 | Prep time: 10 min | | Total time: 10 min |

Nutrition per Serving: Calories: 200, Protein: 3g, Carbohydrates: 15g, Fat: 15g, Fiber: 5g

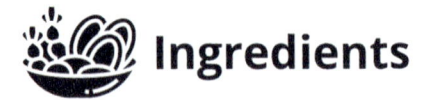

Ingredients

- 2 ripe avocados
- 1/4 cup unsweetened cocoa powder
- 1/4 cup honey or maple syrup (or to taste)
- 1 teaspoon vanilla extract
- Pinch of sea salt
- 1 tablespoon maca powder (optional)
- Fresh berries for serving

Directions

- Cut the avocados in half, remove the pits, and scoop the flesh into a food processor.
- Add the cocoa powder, honey or maple syrup, vanilla extract, sea salt, and maca powder (if using) to the food processor.
- Blend until smooth and creamy, scraping down the sides as needed.
- Taste and adjust sweetness if necessary by adding more honey or maple syrup.
- Divide the mousse into serving dishes and refrigerate for at least 30 minutes to chill.
- Serve topped with fresh berries.

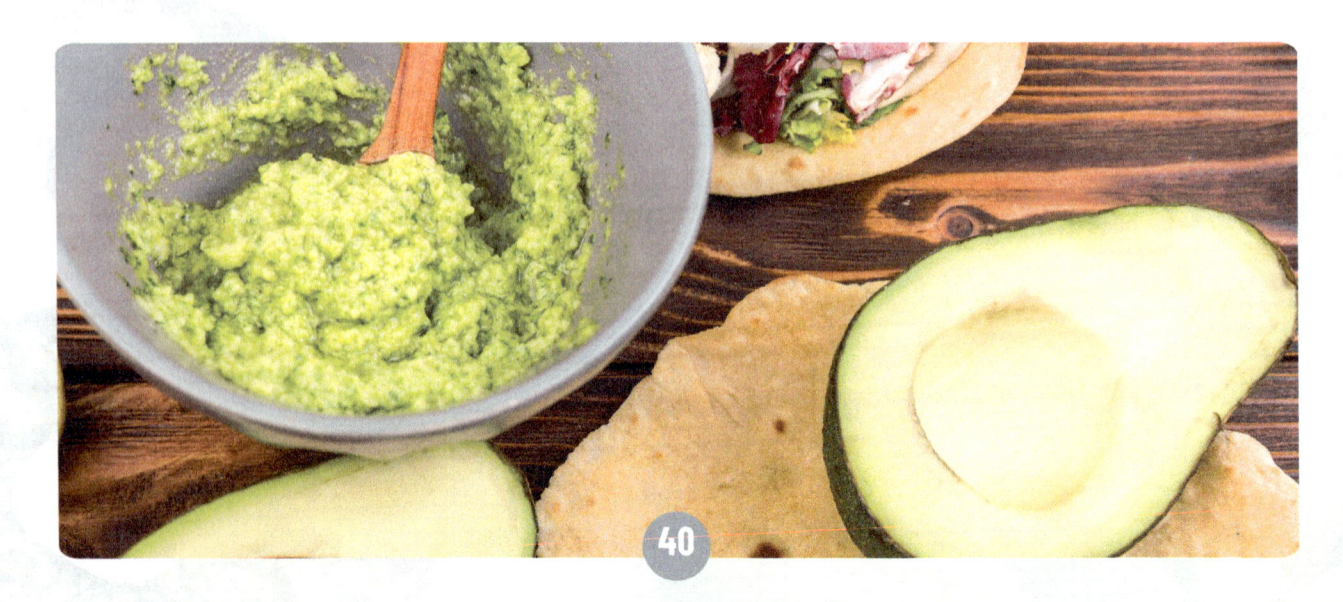

Decadent Delights

\multicolumn{4}{c}{**Chocolate Chip Banana Bread Bars**}
Servings: 12 bars	Prep time: 15 min		Total time: 45 min

Nutrition per Serving: Calories: 150, Protein: 3g, Carbohydrates: 20g, Fat: 7g, Fiber: 3g

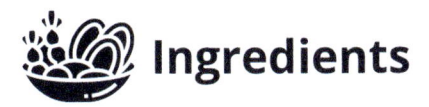

Ingredients

- 2 ripe bananas, mashed
- 1/4 cup honey or maple syrup
- 1/4 cup coconut oil, melted
- 1 teaspoon vanilla extract
- 2 cups almond flour
- 1/2 teaspoon baking soda
- Pinch of salt
- 1/2 cup dark chocolate chips (sugar-free optional)

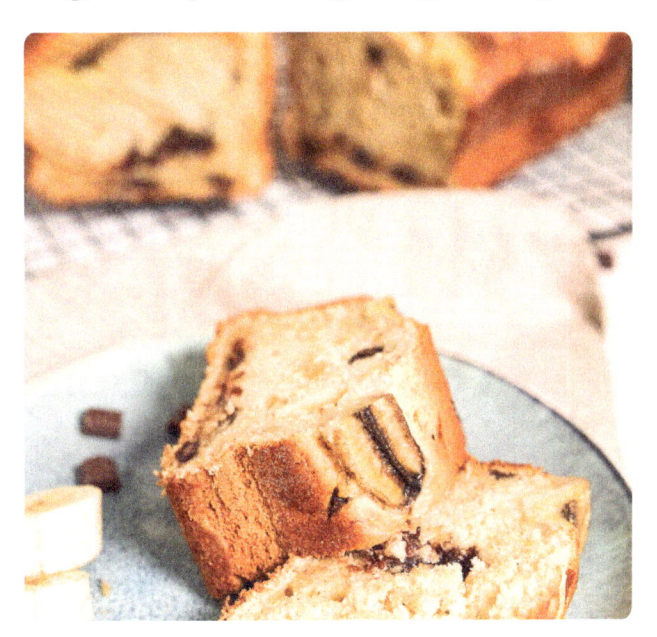

Directions

- Preheat your oven to 350°F (175°C) and grease a baking dish.
- In a large mixing bowl, combine the mashed bananas, honey or maple syrup, melted coconut oil, and vanilla extract.
- Add both the almond flour, baking soda, and salt to the wet ingredients, and then mix properly until well combined.
- Fold in the dark chocolate chips.
- Pour the batter into the prepared baking dish after which you should spread it evenly.
- Bake for 25-30 minutes, or until golden brown and set in the center.
- Allow to cool before slicing into bars. Enjoy as a guilt-free snack or dessert!

Raspberry Chia Seed Pudding Parfaits

Servings: 4 parfaits	Prep time: 10 minutes (+overnight chilling)	10 minutes (+overnight chilling)

Nutrition per Serving: Calories: 180, Protein: 4g, Carbohydrates: 20g, Fat: 10g, Fiber: 7g

Ingredients

- 1 cup unsweetened almond milk
- 1/4 cup chia seeds
- 1 tablespoon honey or maple syrup
- 1 teaspoon vanilla extract
- 1 cup fresh raspberries
- Sliced almonds or shredded coconut for topping (optional)

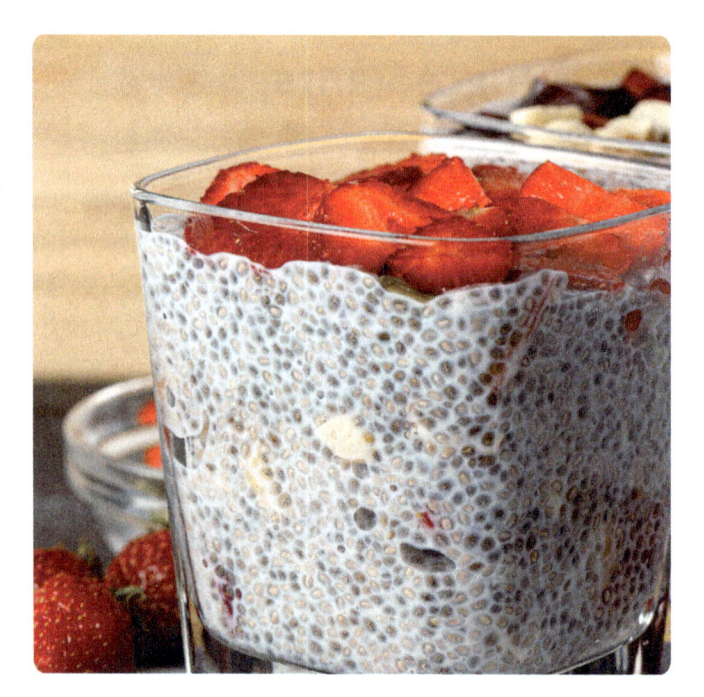

Directions

- In a mixing bowl, whisk together the almond milk, chia seeds, honey or maple syrup, and vanilla extract.
- Cover and refrigerate overnight, or for at least 4 hours, to allow the chia seeds to gel and thicken the pudding.
- Before serving, layer the chia seed pudding and fresh raspberries in serving glasses or jars.
- Top with sliced almonds or shredded coconut for added texture and flavor, if desired.
- Serve chilled and enjoy the creamy, fruity goodness of these guilt-free parfaits!

Nourishing Frozen Treats

Protein-Packed Berry Bliss Nice Cream		
Servings: 4	Prep time: 10 minutes	4 hours (including freezing time)

Nutrition per Serving: Calories: 150, Protein: 5g, Carbohydrates: 20g, Fat: 7g, Fiber: 6g

Ingredients

- 2 ripe bananas, sliced and frozen
- 1 cup mixed berries (such as strawberries, blueberries, raspberries)
- 1/4 cup plain Greek yogurt
- 2 tablespoons almond butter
- 1 tablespoon chia seeds
- 1 teaspoon vanilla extract
- Optional: stevia or erythritol for additional sweetness

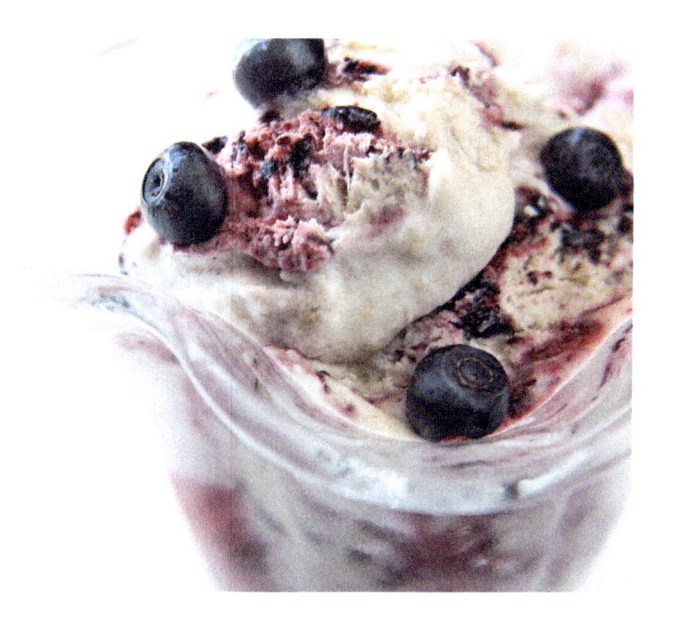

Directions

- In a blender or food processor, combine the frozen banana slices, mixed berries, Greek yogurt, almond butter, chia seeds, and vanilla extract.
- Blend until smooth and creamy, adjusting sweetness with stevia or erythritol if desired.
- Transfer the nice cream mixture into a freezer-safe container and freeze for at least 4 hours, or until firm.
- Serve scoops of protein-packed berry bliss nice cream in bowls or cones, and enjoy the cool, creamy goodness guilt-free!

Superfood Spinach-Berry Popsicles

Servings: 6 popsicles	Prep time: 10 minutes	4 hours (including freezing time)

Nutrition per Serving: Calories: 60, Protein: 2g, Carbohydrates: 10g, Fat: 2g, Fiber: 3g

Ingredients

- 1 cup spinach leaves
- 1 ripe banana
- 1 cup mixed berries (such as strawberries, blueberries, raspberries)
- 1/2 cup unsweetened almond milk
- 1 tablespoon chia seeds
- 1 tablespoon honey or maple syrup
- Optional: a squeeze of lemon juice

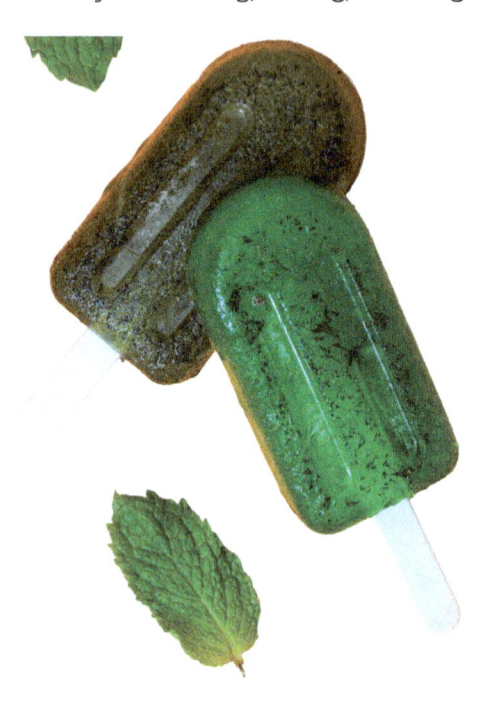

Directions

- In a blender, combine the spinach leaves, banana, mixed berries, almond milk, chia seeds, and honey or maple syrup.
- Add a squeeze of lemon juice for a burst of freshness, if desired.
- Blend until smooth and well combined.
- Pour the mixture into popsicle molds, leaving a little space at the top for expansion.
- Insert popsicle sticks into the molds and freeze for at least 4 hours, or until completely solid.
- To unmold the popsicles, run the molds under warm water for a few seconds and gently pull out the popsicles.
- Enjoy these superfood spinach-berry popsicles as a nutritious and refreshing treat, packed with vitamins, minerals, and antioxidants to support your wellness journey.

CHAPTER 8

PCOS-FRIENDLY BEVERAGES

Quench your thirst and support your wellness journey with hydrating and flavorful beverages tailored to managing PCOS. In this chapter, we explore the importance of staying hydrated and creative ways to infuse flavor into water to keep you refreshed and satisfied.

Hydration Station:

Importance of Staying Hydrated with PCOS
Staying hydrated is crucial for overall health, particularly for individuals managing PCOS.

Here are ten important reasons highlighting the significance of hydration in PCOS management:

1. Regulates Hormonal Balance: Adequate hydration supports the body's ability to maintain hormonal balance, which is essential for managing PCOS symptoms.
2. Supports Metabolism: Proper hydration helps support metabolic function, aiding in weight management and insulin sensitivity, both of which are important considerations for PCOS management.
3. Promotes Digestive Health: Drinking enough water supports healthy digestion and prevents constipation, promoting regular bowel movements and reducing bloating, common concerns for individuals with PCOS.
4. Enhances Detoxification: Hydration supports the body's natural detoxification processes, helping to flush out toxins and waste products that can contribute to inflammation and hormonal imbalances.
5. Improves Skin Health: Adequate hydration helps maintain skin elasticity and hydration, reducing the risk of acne and promoting a clear, radiant complexion often affected by hormonal fluctuations in PCOS.
6. Supports Kidney Function: Proper hydration is essential for kidney health, aiding in the filtration of waste products and preventing kidney stones, a potential complication associated with PCOS.
7. Boosts Energy Levels: Dehydration can lead to fatigue and reduced energy levels, impacting daily activities and exercise performance, which are important for managing PCOS symptoms and promoting overall well-being.
8. Aids in Weight Management: Drinking water before meals can help promote a feeling of fullness, reducing calorie intake and supporting weight management efforts, a key aspect of PCOS management.
9. Regulates Body Temperature: Hydration helps regulate body temperature, preventing overheating and supporting optimal physiological function, particularly during exercise or in hot weather.
10. Improves Mood and Cognitive Function: Dehydration can negatively impact mood and cognitive function, leading to irritability, difficulty concentrating, and mood swings, all of which can affect daily life and PCOS management.

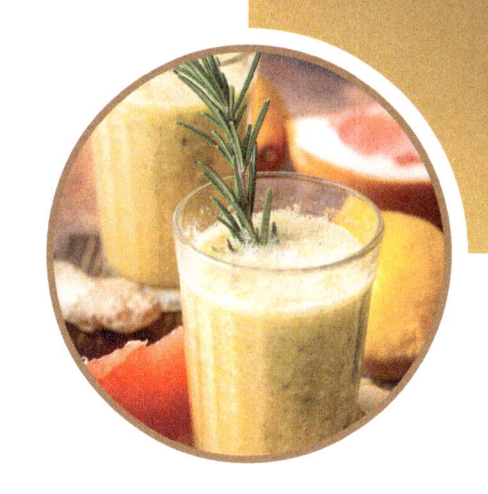

By prioritizing hydration and ensuring adequate fluid intake throughout the day, individuals with PCOS can support their overall health and well-being, effectively managing symptoms and promoting hormonal balance.

Creative Ways to Infuse Flavor into Water

While plain water is essential for hydration, infusing it with natural flavors can make it more enjoyable and enticing.

Here are some creative ways to add flavor to your water:

1. Citrus Infusions: Add slices of lemon, lime, or orange to your water for a refreshing citrus flavor, along with a boost of vitamin C and antioxidants.

2. Herbal Enhancements: Experiment with fresh herbs like mint, basil, or rosemary to infuse your water with aromatic flavors and a hint of natural sweetness.

3. Cucumber Coolness: Thinly slice cucumbers and add them to your water for a crisp and refreshing taste, perfect for staying hydrated on hot days.

4. Berry Burst: Mix in a handful of fresh berries such as strawberries, blueberries, or raspberries for a burst of color and natural sweetness, along with added antioxidants.

5. Tropical Twist: Add chunks of pineapple or slices of mango to your water for a taste of the tropics, along with a hint of natural sweetness and vitamin C.

6. Spa-like Elegance: Create a spa-inspired water by adding cucumber slices, mint leaves, and a splash of lemon or lime juice for a refreshing and revitalizing beverage.

7. Ginger Zing: Grate fresh ginger root and steep it in hot water before cooling for a spicy and invigorating drink, perfect for supporting digestion and reducing inflammation.

8. Fruit Fusion: Mix and match your favorite fruits and herbs to create unique flavor combinations, such as strawberry basil or lemon-lime-mint, for a personalized hydration experience.

Herbal Infusions and Teas

Discover five unique and healthy recipes for homemade tea blends designed to nurture your body and promote overall wellness.

Healing Properties of Herbal Teas for PCOS Symptoms

Herbal teas offer a natural and gentle way to address various PCOS symptoms by harnessing the therapeutic properties of medicinal herbs.

Here are some key healing properties of herbal teas for managing PCOS symptoms:

1. **Hormone Regulation:** Certain herbs like chasteberry (Vitex agnus-castus) and spearmint have been shown to help regulate hormone levels, including testosterone and estrogen, which can be imbalanced in individuals with PCOS.
2. **Insulin Sensitivity:** Herbs such as cinnamon and fenugreek may help improve insulin sensitivity and regulate blood sugar levels, which is beneficial for managing insulin resistance, a common feature of PCOS.
3. **Anti-inflammatory Effects:** Turmeric, ginger, and licorice root possess potent anti-inflammatory properties that can help reduce inflammation associated with PCOS, alleviating symptoms such as pain and bloating.
4. **Digestive Support:** Peppermint and fennel are known for their digestive benefits, helping to soothe gastrointestinal discomfort and promote healthy digestion, which can be compromised in individuals with PCOS.
5. **Stress Reduction:** Adaptogenic herbs like holy basil (tulsi) and ashwagandha can help modulate the body's stress response and promote relaxation, which is important for managing stress-related symptoms of PCOS such as anxiety and mood swings.

Homemade Tea Blends

Hormone Harmony Blend

Servings: 2 cups   Prep time: 5 min   Total time: 10 min

Ingredients

- 1 teaspoon dried spearmint leaves
- 1 teaspoon dried chasteberry (Vitex)
- 1 teaspoon cinnamon chips
- 2 cups water

Benefits: Spearmint, chasteberry, and cinnamon helps to support hormone balance, regulate menstrual cycles, and reduce testosterone levels associated with PCOS.

Directions

- Use a small saucepan to bring water to a boil.
- Add dried spearmint leaves, chasteberry, and cinnamon chips to the boiling water.
- Reduce the heat and then let simmer for about 5 minutes..
- Strain the tea into cups and enjoy warm

Insulin Support Blend

Servings: 2 cups   Prep time: 5 min   Total time: 10 min

Ingredients

- 1 teaspoon fenugreek seeds
- 1 teaspoon cinnamon powder
- 1 teaspoon grated ginger root
- 2 cups water

Benefits: Fenugreek, cinnamon, and ginger work together to improve insulin sensitivity, regulate blood sugar levels, and support metabolic function, making this blend ideal for individuals managing insulin resistance associated with PCOS.

Directions

- Use a small saucepan to bring water to a boil.
- Add fenugreek seeds, cinnamon powder, and grated ginger root to the boiling water.
- Reduce the heat and then let simmer for about 5 minutes.
- Strain the tea into cups and enjoy warm.

Anti-inflammatory Elixir

Servings: 2 cups   Prep time: 5 min   Total time: 10 min

Ingredients

- 1 teaspoon turmeric powder
- 1 teaspoon sliced ginger root
- 1 teaspoon licorice root
- 2 cups water

Benefits: Turmeric, ginger, and licorice root possess potent anti-inflammatory properties that can help reduce inflammation associated with PCOS, alleviating symptoms such as pain and bloating.

Directions

- Use a small saucepan to bring water to a boil.
- Add turmeric powder, sliced ginger root, and licorice root to the boiling water.
- Reduce the heat and give it time to simmer for 5 minutes.
- Strain the tea into cups and enjoy warm.

Digestive Ease Blend

Servings: 2 cups   Prep time: 5 min   Total time: 10 min

Ingredients

- 1 teaspoon dried peppermint leaves
- 1 teaspoon fennel seeds
- 1 teaspoon chamomile flowers
- 2 cups water

Benefits: Peppermint, fennel, and chamomile support digestive health, soothing gastrointestinal discomfort and promoting regular bowel movements, which can be compromised in individuals with PCOS.

Directions

- Use a small saucepan to bring water to a boil.
- Add dried peppermint leaves, fennel seeds, and chamomile flowers to the boiling water.
- Reduce the heat and let it simmer for about 5 minutes.
- Strain the tea into cups and enjoy warm.

Stress Relief Soother

Servings: 2 cups   Prep time: 5 min   Total time: 10 min

Ingredients

- 1 teaspoon dried holy basil (tulsi) leaves
- 1 teaspoon ashwagandha root
- 1 teaspoon dried lemon balm leaves
- 2 cups water

Benefits: Holy basil, ashwagandha, and lemon balm help modulate the body's stress response, promoting relaxation and reducing symptoms of anxiety and mood swings commonly associated with PCOS.

Directions

- Use a small saucepan to bring water to a boil.
- Add dried holy basil leaves, ashwagandha root, and dried lemon balm leaves to the boiling water.
- Reduce the heat and then let simmer for about 5 minutes.
- Strain the tea into cups and enjoy warm.

Liver Love Infusion

Servings: 2 cups   Prep time: 5 min   Total time: 10 min

Ingredients

- 1 teaspoon dried dandelion root
- 1 teaspoon milk thistle seeds
- 1 teaspoon dried burdock root
- 2 cups water

Benefits: Dandelion root, milk thistle, and burdock root support liver detoxification, aiding in the elimination of toxins and promoting hormonal balance, essential for individuals managing PCOS.

Directions

- Get a small saucepan to bring water to a boil.
- Add dried dandelion root, milk thistle seeds, and dried burdock root to the boiling water.
- Reduce the heat and then let simmer for about 5 minutes.
- Strain the tea into cups and enjoy warm.

Smoothie and Juice Boosters

Berry Blast Smoothie Booster

Servings: 1 Prep time: 5 min Total time: 10 min

<u>Nutrition per Serving:</u> Calories: 200, Protein: 15g, Carbohydrates: 22g, Fat: 7g, Fiber: 8g

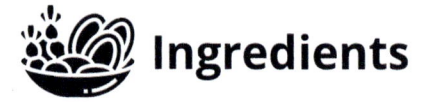

Ingredients

- 1 tablespoon ground flaxseed
- 1 tablespoon chia seeds
- 1/2 cup mixed berries (strawberries, blueberries, raspberries)
- 1/2 cup spinach leaves
- 1/2 cup unsweetened almond milk
- 1/2 cup Greek yogurt (optional)
- Optional: 1 scoop protein powder

Directions

- Combine all ingredients in a blender.
- Blend until smooth and creamy.
- Pour it into a glass and serve.

Green Goddess Juice Booster

Servings: 1 Prep time: 5 min Total time: 10 min

<u>Nutrition per Serving:</u> Calories: 150, Protein: 7g, Carbohydrates: 30g, Fat: 1g, Fiber: 10g

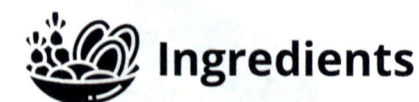

Ingredients

- 1 tablespoon wheatgrass powder
- 1 tablespoon spirulina powder
- 1 green apple, cored and chopped
- 1/2 cucumber, chopped
- 1/2 lemon, juiced
- 1 cup spinach leaves
- 1/2 cup water or coconut water
- Ice cubes (optional)

Directions

- Put all the ingredients together in a juicer or blender.
- Blend or juice until smooth.
- Strain the juice if desired.
- Pour over ice and serve immediately.

Tropical Turmeric Smoothie Booster

Servings: 1 | Prep time: 5 min | Total time: 10 min

Nutrition per Serving: Calories: 250, Protein: 7g, Carbohydrates: 55g, Fat: 1g, Fiber: 8g

Ingredients

- 1 tablespoon ground turmeric
- 1 tablespoon ground ginger
- 1/2 cup pineapple chunks
- 1/2 cup mango chunks
- 1/2 banana
- 1/2 cup coconut water
- 1/4 cup coconut or Greek yogurt

Directions

- Blend all ingredients until smooth.
- Garnish with turmeric or ginger if desired.
- Serve immediately.

Creamy Cocoa Protein Shake

Servings: 1 | Prep time: 5 min | Total time: 10 min

Nutrition per Serving: Calories: 250, Protein: 25g, Carbohydrates: 22g, Fat: 9g, Fiber: 6g

Ingredients

- 1 tablespoon cocoa powder (unsweetened)
- 1 tablespoon almond butter
- 1/2 banana
- 1/2 cup unsweetened almond milk
- 1/2 cup Greek yogurt
- 1 scoop protein powder (chocolate-flavored, optional)

Directions

- Combine all ingredients in a blender.
- Blend until smooth and creamy.
- Transfer into a glass and serve promptly.

Golden Glow Turmeric Latte

Servings: 1   Prep time: 5 min   Total time: 10 min

Nutrition per Serving: Calories: 100, Protein: 1g, Carbohydrates: 20g, Fat: 2g, Fiber: 2g

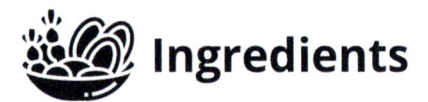

Ingredients

- 1 tablespoon ground turmeric
- 1/2 teaspoon ground cinnamon
- Pinch of black pepper
- 1 tablespoon honey (or maple syrup for vegan option)
- 1 cup unsweetened almond milk
- 1/2 teaspoon vanilla extract

Directions

- Warm the almond milk in a small saucepan over medium heat, ensuring it doesn't reach boiling point.
- Whisk in turmeric, cinnamon, black pepper, honey (or maple syrup), and vanilla extract until well combined.
- Pour into a mug and savor it while it's warm

Berry Beet Detox Juice

Servings: 1   Prep time: 5 min   Total time: 10 min

Nutrition per Serving: Calories: 80, Protein: 2g, Carbohydrates: 18g, Fat: 0.5g, Fiber: 4g

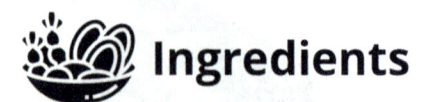

Ingredients

- 1 small beet, peeled and chopped
- 1/2 cup mixed berries (strawberries, blueberries, raspberries)
- 1/2 cucumber, chopped
- 1/2 lemon, juiced
- 1/2 inch ginger root, peeled
- 1 cup water or coconut water
- Ice cubes (optional)

Directions

- Combine all ingredients in a juicer or blender.
- Blend or juice until smooth.
- Strain the juice if desired.
- Pour over ice and serve immediately.

CHAPTER 9

VEGETARIAN AND VEGAN ENTRÉES

Plant-Powered Protein Recipes

Quinoa Stuffed Bell Peppers

Servings: 4 | Prep time: 15 min | Cook time: 30 min | Total time: 45 min

<u>Nutrition per Serving:</u> Calories: 320, Protein: 14g, Carbohydrates: 63g, Fat: 2g, Fiber: 14g

Ingredients

- 4 bell peppers, cut in half with seeds removed
- 1 cup quinoa, rinsed
- 2 cups vegetable broth
- 1 can (15 ounces) of black beans, drained and thoroughly rinsed
- 1 cup corn kernels (fresh or frozen)
- 1 cup cherry tomatoes, halved
- 1/2 cup red onion, diced
- 2 cloves garlic, minced
- 1 teaspoon cumin
- 1 teaspoon chili powder
- Salt and pepper to taste
- Fresh cilantro, for garnish

Protein-Rich Plant Foods:
Incorporate protein-rich plant foods like quinoa, black beans, and corn into this hearty vegetarian dish to support balanced nutrition and provide essential nutrients for managing PCOS.

Directions

- Preheat oven to 375°F (190°C).
- In a saucepan, mix together quinoa and vegetable broth. Bring to a boil, then reduce heat, cover, and simmer for 15-20 minutes, or until quinoa is cooked and liquid is absorbed.
- In a large mixing bowl, combine cooked quinoa, black beans, corn, cherry tomatoes, red onion, minced garlic, cumin, chili powder, salt, and pepper. Mix well.
- Arrange halved bell peppers in a baking dish.
- Use a spoon to fill each pepper half with the quinoa mixture.
- Cover the baking dish with foil and bake for 25-30 minutes, or until peppers are tender.
- Serve hot, garnished with fresh cilantro.

Lentil and Vegetable Stir-Fry

| Servings: 4 | Prep time: 15 min | Cook time: 20 min | Total time: 35 min |

Nutrition per Serving: Calories: 290, Protein: 14g, Carbohydrates: 41g, Fat: 9g, Fiber: 11g

Ingredients

- 1 cup green lentils, rinsed
- 2 cups vegetable broth
- 2 tablespoons olive oil
- 1 onion, thinly sliced
- 2 carrots, julienned
- 1 bell pepper, thinly sliced
- 2 cups broccoli florets
- 3 cloves garlic, minced
- 1 tablespoon ginger, grated
- 1/4 cup low-sodium soy sauce or tamari
- 1 tablespoon sesame oil
- 2 tablespoons rice vinegar
- 1 tablespoon of maple syrup or honey (if desired)
- Already cooked brown rice or quinoa, for serving
- Sesame seeds and scallions (green onions) for garnishing

Protein-Rich Plant Foods: Lentils serve as an excellent plant-based protein source in this flavorful stir-fry, while a variety of colorful vegetables provide essential nutrients and fiber for optimal health.

Directions

- In a saucepan, combine green lentils and vegetable broth. Bring to a boil, then reduce heat, cover, and simmer for 15-20 minutes, or until lentils are tender.
- Warm olive oil in a sizable skillet or wok on medium-high heat. Add sliced onion, julienned carrots, and sliced bell pepper. Stir-fry for 3-4 minutes until vegetables start to soften.
- Add broccoli florets, minced garlic, and grated ginger to the skillet. Continue to stir-fry for another 2-3 minutes.
- In a small bowl, whisk together soy sauce or tamari, sesame oil, rice vinegar, and maple syrup or honey (if using). Drizzle the sauce onto the vegetables in the skillet.
- Add cooked lentils to the skillet and toss everything together until well combined and heated through.
- Serve the lentil and vegetable stir-fry hot over cooked brown rice or quinoa.
- Add sesame seeds and sliced green onions as garnish prior to serving.

Chickpea and Vegetable Curry

Servings: 4	Prep time: 15 min	Cook time: 20 min	Total time: 35 min

<u>Nutrition per Serving:</u> Calories: 320, Protein: 6g, Carbohydrates: 30g, Fat: 20g, Fiber: 8g

Ingredients

- 1 tablespoon coconut oil
- 1 onion, diced
- 3 cloves garlic, minced
- 1 tablespoon fresh ginger, grated
- 2 tablespoons curry powder
- 1 teaspoon ground turmeric
- 1 teaspoon ground cumin
- 1 can (15 ounces) of chickpeas, drained and thoroughly rinsed
- 1 can (14 oz) coconut milk
- 2 cups cauliflower florets
- 1 cup of diced tomatoes, whether fresh or canned
- 1 cup spinach leaves
- Salt and pepper to taste
- Already cooked brown rice or quinoa, for serving
- Fresh cilantro, for garnish

Protein-Rich Plant Foods: Chickpeas are a rich source of plant-based protein in this vibrant curry, while cauliflower, spinach, and tomatoes provide an array of vitamins, minerals, and antioxidants essential for supporting overall health and managing PCOS symptoms

Directions

- Warm coconut oil in a large skillet or pot on medium heat. Then, add diced onion, minced garlic, and grated ginger. Cook until onion is soft and translucent, about 3-4 minutes.
- Stir in curry powder, ground turmeric, and ground cumin. Cook for another minute until fragrant.
- Add chickpeas, coconut milk, cauliflower florets, and diced tomatoes to the skillet. Stir to combine.
- Cover and simmer for 15-20 minutes, or until cauliflower is tender and flavors are well blended.
- Stir in spinach leaves and cook until wilted, about 2-3 minutes. Season with salt and pepper to your liking.
- Serve the chickpea and vegetable curry hot over cooked brown rice or quinoa.
- Garnish with fresh cilantro before serving.

Eggplant and Lentil Moussaka

Servings: 6 | Prep time: 30 min | Cook time: 50 min | Total time: 1 hour 20 minutes

Nutrition per Serving: Calories: 280, Protein: 15g, Carbohydrates: 40g, Fat: 8g, Fiber: 12g

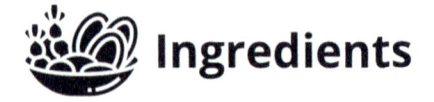

Ingredients

- 2 large eggplants, sliced lengthwise
- 1 cup green lentils, rinsed
- 2 cups vegetable broth
- 2 tablespoons olive oil
- 1 onion, diced
- 3 cloves garlic, minced
- 1 red bell pepper, diced
- 1 zucchini, diced
- 1 can (14 oz) diced tomatoes
- 1 tablespoon tomato paste
- 1 teaspoon dried oregano
- 1 teaspoon dried basil
- Salt and pepper to taste
- 1 cup plain Greek yogurt or dairy-free yogurt alternative
- 1/4 cup grated Parmesan cheese or vegan cheese alternative
- Fresh parsley, for garnish

Protein-Rich Plant Foods: Green lentils and Greek yogurt provide ample plant-based protein in this comforting and nutritious vegetarian moussaka, offering a satisfying meal option for women with PCOS.

Directions

- Preheat oven to 375°F (190°C).
- Arrange eggplant slices on a baking sheet covered with parchment paper. Bake for 15-20 minutes, or until tender.
- Remove from oven and set aside.
- In a saucepan, combine green lentils and vegetable broth. Bring to a boil, then reduce heat, cover, and simmer for 15-20 minutes, or until lentils are tender.
- In a sizable skillet, warm olive oil over medium heat. Add diced onion and minced garlic, and cook until softened, about 3-4 minutes.
- Add diced bell pepper and zucchini to the skillet, and cook for another 5 minutes, or until vegetables are tender.
- Stir in diced tomatoes, tomato paste, dried oregano, dried basil, cooked lentils, salt, and pepper.
- Simmer for 10 minutes, allowing flavors to meld together.

Spinach and Chickpea Curry

| Servings: 4 | Prep time: 10 min | Cook time: 25 min | Total time: 35 min |

Nutrition per Serving: Calories: 280, Protein: 10g, Carbohydrates: 30g, Fat: 14g, Fiber: 8g

Ingredients

- 1 tablespoon olive oil
- 1 onion, diced
- 3 cloves garlic, minced
- 1 tablespoon fresh ginger, grated
- 2 tablespoons curry powder
- 1 teaspoon ground cumin
- 1 teaspoon ground coriander
- 1 can (15 ounces) chickpeas, drained and washed
- 1 can (14 oz) diced tomatoes
- 1 can (14 oz) coconut milk
- 4 cups fresh spinach leaves
- Salt and pepper to taste
- Cooked brown rice or quinoa, for serving
- Fresh cilantro, for garnish

Protein-Rich Plant Foods: Chickpeas and spinach are excellent sources of plant-based protein in this flavorful curry, providing essential nutrients for managing PCOS symptoms while offering a delicious meatless meal option

Directions

- Warm olive oil in a spacious skillet on medium heat. Add diced onion and cook until translucent, about 3-4 minutes.
- Mix in minced garlic and grated ginger, then cook for an additional minute until aromatic.
- Add curry powder, ground cumin, and ground coriander to the skillet, and cook for 1-2 minutes to toast the spices.
- Add chickpeas, diced tomatoes, and coconut milk to the skillet. Stir to combine.
- Bring the mixture to a simmer and let it cook for 15 minutes, allowing the flavors to meld together.
- Stir in fresh spinach leaves and cook until wilted, about 2-3 minutes.
- Add salt and pepper to your preference..
- Serve the spinach and chickpea curry hot over cooked brown rice or quinoa.
- Garnish with fresh cilantro before serving.

Mushroom and Lentil Shepherd's Pie

Servings: 6	Prep time: 20 min	Cook time: 40 min	Total time: 1 hour

<u>Nutrition per Serving:</u> Calories: 320, Protein: 12g, Carbohydrates: 55g, Fat: 6g, Fiber: 14g

Ingredients

- 1 tablespoon olive oil
- 1 onion, diced
- 2 carrots, diced
- 2 celery stalks, diced
- 2 cloves garlic, minced
- 8 oz mushrooms, sliced
- 1 cup green lentils, rinsed
- 2 cups vegetable broth
- 2 tablespoons tomato paste
- 1 teaspoon dried thyme
- 1 teaspoon dried rosemary
- Salt and pepper to taste
- 4 cups of prepared mashed potatoes
- Fresh parsley, for garnish

Protein-Rich Plant Foods: Green lentils provide a hearty source of plant-based protein in this comforting shepherd's pie, while mushrooms add depth of flavor and essential nutrients for supporting hormone balance and managing PCOS symptoms

Directions

- Preheat oven to 375°F (190°C). Lightly grease a 9x13-inch baking dish.
- Warm the olive oil in a spacious skillet over medium heat. Add diced onion, carrots, and celery. Cook until vegetables are softened, about 5 minutes.
- Add minced garlic and sliced mushrooms to the skillet. Cook until mushrooms are tender and any liquid has evaporated, about 5-7 minutes.
- Stir in rinsed green lentils, vegetable broth, tomato paste, dried thyme, dried rosemary, salt, and pepper. Bring to a simmer, then reduce heat and let it simmer for 20-25 minutes, or until lentils are cooked and most of the liquid is absorbed.
- Transfer the lentil and mushroom mixture to the prepared baking dish, spreading it out evenly.
- Spread the mashed potatoes over the lentil mixture, covering it completely.
- Bake in the preheated oven for 20-25 minutes, or until the top is golden brown and the filling is bubbly.
- Take it out of the oven and allow it to cool for a bit before serving.
- Garnish with fresh parsley before serving.

Flavorful Grain-Based Dishes

Mediterranean Farro Salad

Servings: 4	Prep time: 15 min	Cook time: 25 min	Total time: 40 min

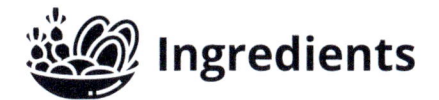

Nutrition per Serving: Calories: 280, Protein: 8g, Carbohydrates: 50g, Fat: 7g, Fiber: 10g

Ingredients

- 1 cup farro, rinsed
- 2 cups vegetable broth
- 1 tablespoon olive oil
- 1 red onion, thinly sliced
- 1 red bell pepper, diced
- 1 yellow bell pepper, diced
- 1 cup cherry tomatoes, halved
- 1/2 cup Kalamata olives, pitted and halved
- 1/4 cup fresh parsley, chopped
- 1/4 cup fresh basil, chopped
- 1/4 cup crumbled feta cheese (optional)
- Salt and pepper to taste
- Lemon wedges, for serving

Healthy Tip: Farro is a nutrient-rich whole grain that's high in fiber and protein, making it a great option for women with PCOS looking to support their health goals.

Directions

- In a saucepan, combine farro and vegetable broth. Bring to a boil, then reduce heat and simmer for 20-25 minutes, or until farro is tender.
- Next, warm up some olive oil in a skillet on medium heat. Add sliced red onion and cook until caramelized, about 10-12 minutes.
- In a large bowl, combine cooked farro, caramelized red onion, diced bell peppers, cherry tomatoes, Kalamata olives, chopped parsley, and chopped basil. Toss to combine.
- If using, sprinkle crumbled feta cheese over the salad. Season with salt and pepper to taste.
- Serve the Mediterranean farro salad at room temperature or chilled, with lemon wedges on the side.

Vegetable Stir-Fry with Brown Rice

| Servings: 4 | Prep time: 15 min | Cook time: 15 min | Total time: 30 min |

Nutrition per Serving: Calories: 280, Protein: 8g, Carbohydrates: 55g, Fat: 4g, Fiber: 8g

Ingredients

- 1 cup brown rice, rinsed
- 2 cups water
- 2 tablespoons of soy sauce (or tamari for a gluten-free alternative)
- 1 tablespoon rice vinegar
- 1 tablespoon sesame oil
- 2 cloves garlic, minced
- 1 tablespoon fresh ginger, grated
- 1 red bell pepper, sliced
- 1 yellow bell pepper, sliced
- 1 cup broccoli florets
- 1 cup snap peas
- 1 medium carrot, julienned
- 1 cup mushrooms, sliced
- 2 green onions, chopped
- Sesame seeds, for garnish (optional)

Healthy Tip: Load up on colorful vegetables to boost your intake of vitamins, minerals, and antioxidants, supporting overall health and wellbeing, particularly important for women managing PCOS.

Directions

- In a saucepan, combine brown rice and water. Bring to a boil, then reduce heat to low, cover, and simmer for 40-45 minutes, or until rice is cooked and water is absorbed.
- In a small bowl, whisk together soy sauce, rice vinegar, and sesame oil to make the sauce. Set aside.
- Heat a sizable skillet or wok on medium-high heat before using. Once heated, add minced garlic and grated ginger, and cook for approximately 1 minute until they become fragrant.
- Add sliced bell peppers, broccoli florets, snap peas, julienned carrot, and sliced mushrooms to the skillet. Stir-fry for 5-6 minutes, or until vegetables are tender-crisp.
- Drizzle the sauce onto the vegetables in the skillet and gently mix until they are evenly coated. Cook for an additional 2-3 minutes.
- Serve the vegetable stir-fry over cooked brown rice, garnished with chopped green onions and sesame seeds if desired.

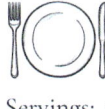

Vegetable and Chickpea Coconut Curry

| Servings: 4 | Prep time: 15 min | Cook time: 25 min | Total time: 40 min |

Nutrition per Serving: Calories: 320, Protein: 10g, Carbohydrates: 40g, Fat: 15g, Fiber: 12g

Ingredients

- 1 tablespoon coconut oil
- 1 onion, diced
- 2 cloves garlic, minced
- 1 tablespoon fresh ginger, grated
- 1 tablespoon curry powder
- 1 teaspoon ground turmeric
- 1 teaspoon ground cumin
- 1 can (14 oz) coconut milk
- 1 can (14 oz) diced tomatoes
- 1 can (15 oz) chickpeas, drained and rinsed
- 2 cups cauliflower florets
- 1 cup green beans, trimmed
- Salt and pepper to taste
- Fresh cilantro, for garnish
- Cooked brown rice or quinoa, for serving

Healthy Tip: Coconut milk adds richness to the curry while providing healthy fats, and chickpeas offer plant-based protein and fiber, making this dish both flavorful and satisfying for women managing PCOS.

Directions

- In a large skillet or pot, heat coconut oil over medium heat. Add diced onion and cook until softened, about 3-4 minutes.
- Add minced garlic and grated ginger to the mixture, stirring well, and continue cooking for one more minute until the aroma becomes fragrant.
- Add curry powder, ground turmeric, and ground cumin to the skillet. Toast the spices for 1-2 minutes while cooking.
- Pour in coconut milk and diced tomatoes, and stir to combine. Bring the mixture to a simmer.
- Add drained chickpeas, cauliflower florets, and green beans to the skillet. Stir to coat the vegetables in the curry sauce.
- Allow the curry to simmer, covered, for 15-20 minutes or until the vegetables have reached desired tenderness.
- Season with salt and pepper to taste.
- Serve the vegetable and chickpea coconut curry hot over cooked brown rice or quinoa.
- Garnish with fresh cilantro before serving.

Dairy-Free Delights

Creamy Avocado Pasta

| Servings: 4 | Prep time: 15 min | Cook time: 10 min | Total time: 25 min |

Nutrition per Serving: Calories: 380, Protein: 9g, Carbohydrates: 49g, Fat: 18g, Fiber: 7g

Ingredients

- 12 ounces spaghetti (gluten-free if needed)
- 2 ripe avocados, peeled and pitted
- 1/4 cup fresh basil leaves
- 2 cloves garlic
- 2 tablespoons lemon juice
- 2 tablespoons olive oil
- Salt and pepper to taste
- Cherry tomatoes, halved, for garnish
- Fresh basil leaves, for garnish

Directions

- Cook spaghetti according to package instructions. Drain and set aside.
- In a food processor or blender, combine avocados, basil leaves, garlic, lemon juice, and olive oil. Blend until smooth and creamy.
- Season avocado sauce with salt and pepper to taste.
- Toss cooked spaghetti with the creamy avocado sauce until evenly coated.
- Serve pasta hot or at room temperature, garnished with cherry tomatoes and fresh basil leaves.

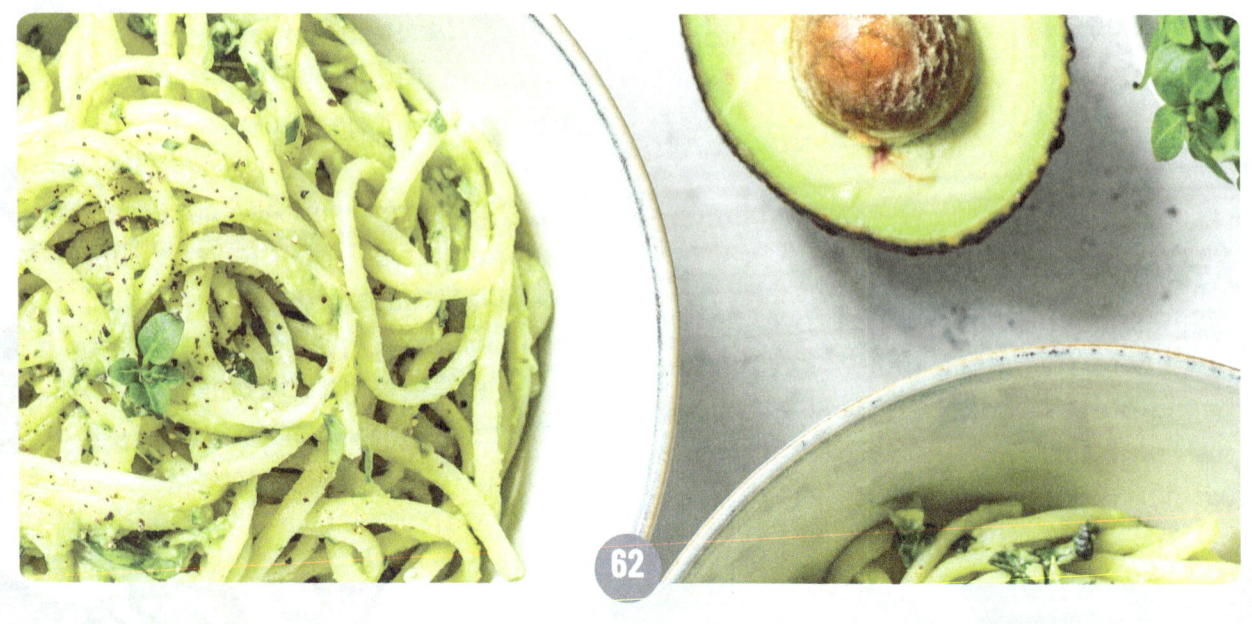

Coconut Curry Lentil Soup

| Servings: 6 | Prep time: 10 min | Cook time: 30 min | Total time: 40 min |

<u>Nutrition per Serving:</u> Calories: 290, Protein: 10g, Carbohydrates: 30g, Fat: 15g, Fiber: 8g

Ingredients

- 1 tablespoon coconut oil
- 1 onion, diced
- 2 carrots, diced
- 2 celery stalks, diced
- 3 cloves garlic, minced
- 1 tablespoon grated fresh ginger
- 1 tablespoon curry powder
- 1 teaspoon ground turmeric
- 1 cup dried red lentils, rinsed
- 4 cups vegetable broth
- 1 can (14 oz) coconut milk
- 2 cups baby spinach
- Salt and pepper to taste
- Fresh cilantro, for garnish
- Lime wedges, for serving

Directions

- Warm the coconut oil in a sizable pot on medium heat. Add diced onion, carrots, and celery. Cook the vegetables until they become tender, approximately 5 minutes.
- Stir in minced garlic, grated ginger, curry powder, and ground turmeric. Cook for another minute until fragrant.
- Add rinsed red lentils and vegetable broth to the pot. Bring to a boil, then reduce heat and simmer for 15-20 minutes, or until lentils are tender.
- Stir in coconut milk and baby spinach. Cook for an additional 5 minutes until spinach is wilted.
- Season the soup with salt and pepper to suit your taste.
- Ladle soup into bowls and garnish with fresh cilantro. Provide lime wedges on the side for serving.

Healthy Tip: Coconut milk adds creaminess to this flavorful lentil soup without the need for dairy, making it a satisfying and nourishing meal for those with dairy sensitivities.

Dairy-Free Pesto Zoodles

| Servings: 2 | Prep time: 15 min | | Total time: 15 min |

Nutrition per Serving: Calories: 320, Protein: 6g, Carbohydrates: 12g, Fat: 28g, Fiber: 4g

Ingredients

- 2 large zucchinis, spiralized into noodles
- 1 cup fresh basil leaves
- 1/4 cup pine nuts
- 2 cloves garlic
- 2 tablespoons nutritional yeast
- 2 tablespoons lemon juice
- 3 tablespoons olive oil
- Salt and pepper to taste
- Cherry tomatoes, halved, for garnish
- Fresh basil leaves, for garnish

Healthy Tip: Nutritional yeast adds a cheesy flavor to the dairy-free pesto sauce, making it a delicious alternative to traditional pesto for those with dairy sensitivities.

Directions

- Transform the zucchinis into noodle-like strands by using either a spiralizer or a julienne peeler. Set aside.
- In a food processor, combine fresh basil leaves, pine nuts, garlic, nutritional yeast, and lemon juice. Pulse until ingredients are finely chopped.
- While the food processor is running, drizzle in the olive oil until a smooth pesto sauce forms. Season with salt and pepper to taste.
- In a large skillet over medium heat, add the zucchini noodles and cook for 2-3 minutes until just softened.
- Add the dairy-free pesto sauce to the skillet with the zucchini noodles and toss to coat evenly.
- Serve the pesto zoodles hot, garnished with cherry tomatoes and fresh basil leaves

Dairy-Free Spinach and Mushroom Risotto

Servings: 4	Prep time: 10 min	Cook time: 30 min	Total time: 40 min

Nutrition per Serving: Calories: 270, Protein: 5g, Carbohydrates: 46g, Fat: 6g, Fiber: 3g

Ingredients

- 1 tablespoon olive oil
- 1 onion, diced
- 2 cloves garlic, minced
- 8 ounces mushrooms, sliced
- 1 cup Arborio rice
- 1/2 cup dry white wine (optional)
- 3 cups vegetable broth
- 2 cups baby spinach
- 1/4 cup nutritional yeast
- Salt and pepper to taste
- Fresh parsley, for garnish

Healthy Tip: Nutritional yeast adds a cheesy flavor to this dairy-free risotto while providing a boost of B vitamins, making it a nutritious and satisfying dish for those with dairy sensitivities.

Directions

- Heat olive oil in a sizable skillet or pot over medium heat. Incorporate diced onion and cook until it turns soft, which usually takes about 5 minutes.
- Stir in minced garlic and sliced mushrooms. Cook for another 5 minutes until mushrooms are golden brown.
- Add Arborio rice to the skillet and cook for 1-2 minutes until lightly toasted.
- If using, pour in dry white wine and stir until absorbed by the rice.
- Gradually add vegetable broth to the skillet, 1/2 cup at a time, stirring frequently and allowing the liquid to absorb before adding more. Continue until the rice is creamy and tender, about 20-25 minutes.
- Stir in baby spinach and nutritional yeast, and cook for another 2-3 minutes until spinach is wilted and nutritional yeast is incorporated.
- Season risotto with salt and pepper to taste.
- Serve the dairy-free spinach and mushroom risotto hot, garnished with fresh parsley.

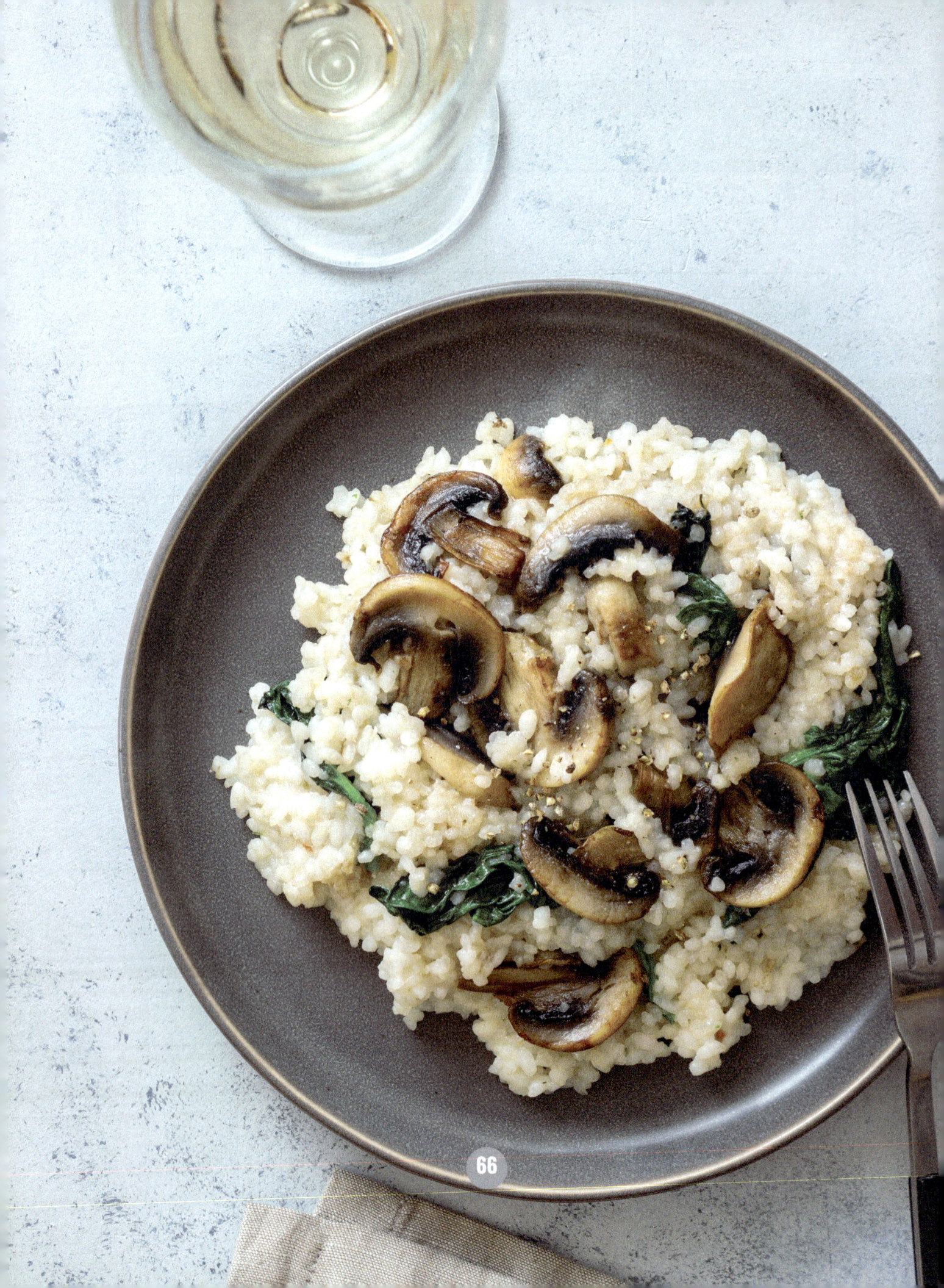

CHAPTER 10

FISH AND SEAFOOD ENTRÉES

Salmon with Lemon Dill Sauce

| Servings: 4 | Prep time: 10 min | Cook time: 15 min | Total time: 25 min |

Nutrition per Serving: Calories: 280, Protein: 34g, Sodium: 75mg, Carbohydrates: 1g, Fat: 15g

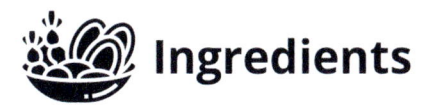

Ingredients

- 4 salmon fillets
- 2 tablespoons olive oil
- 1 tablespoon fresh dill, chopped
- 1 lemon, juiced and zested
- Salt and pepper to taste

Benefits of Omega-3 Fatty Acids: Omega-3 fatty acids found in salmon promote hormone balance and reduce inflammation, helping to alleviate PCOS symptoms.

Directions

- Preheat the oven to 400°F (200°C).
- Arrange the salmon fillets on a baking sheet covered with parchment paper.
- Drizzle olive oil over the fillets and season with salt, pepper, and half of the lemon zest.
- Bake for about 12-15 minutes until salmon is well cooked and flakes easily with a fork.
- In a small bowl, mix lemon juice, remaining lemon zest, and chopped dill to make the sauce.
- Serve salmon hot with lemon dill sauce drizzled on top.

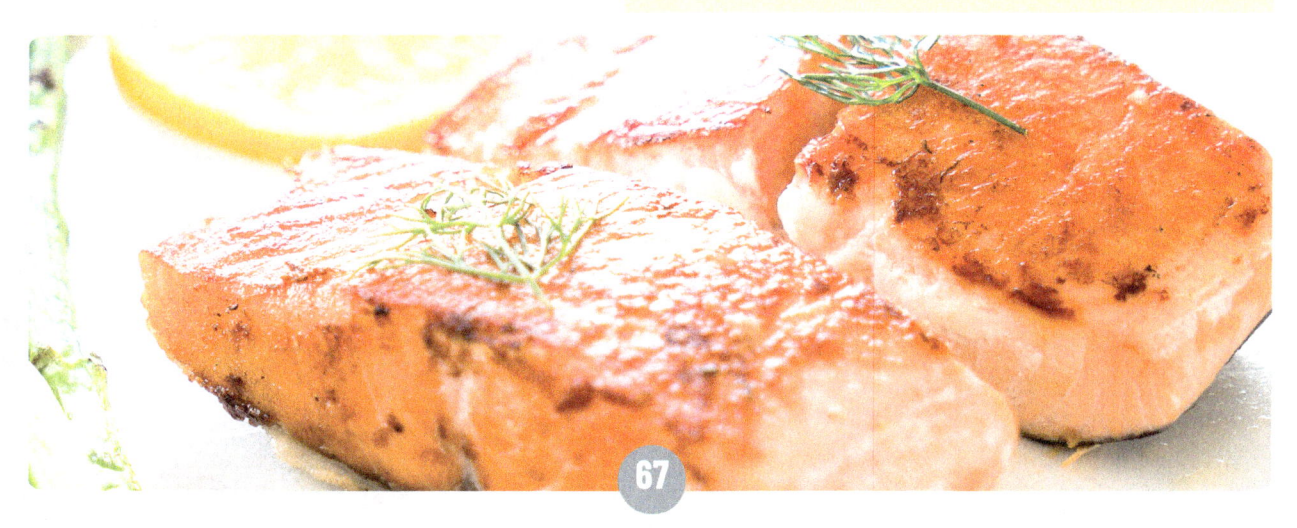

Miso Glazed Cod

Servings: 4,   Prep Time: 10 min   Cook Time: 15 min,   Total Time: 25 min

Nutrition per Serving: Calories: 180, Protein: 26g, Sodium: 650mg, Carbohydrates: 11g, Fat: 3g

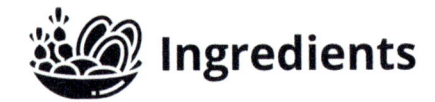

Ingredients

- 4 cod fillets
- 3 tablespoons white miso paste
- 2 tablespoons honey
- 1 tablespoon rice vinegar
- 1 tablespoon soy sauce (or tamari for gluten-free)
- 1 teaspoon sesame oil
- Sesame seeds and diced green onions for garnishing.

Benefits of Omega-3 Fatty Acids: The omega-3 fatty acids in cod contribute to hormone balance and may help reduce insulin resistance in women with PCOS.

Directions

- Preheat the oven to 400°F (200°C).
- In a small bowl, whisk together miso paste, honey, rice vinegar, soy sauce, and sesame oil to make the glaze.
- Place cod fillets on a baking sheet covered with parchment paper.
- Brush the miso glaze over the cod fillets, covering them evenly.
- Bake for about 12-15 minutes until cod is well cooked and flakes easily with a fork.
- Add sesame seeds and chopped green onions as a garnish just before serving.

Shrimp and Avocado Salad

Servings: 2,   Prep Time: 15 min   Cook Time: 5 min,   Total Time: 20 min

Nutrition per Serving: Calories: 320, Protein: 25g, Sodium: 300mg, Carbohydrates: 15g, Fat: 20g

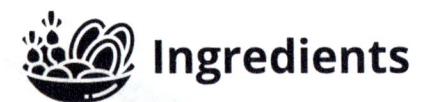

Ingredients

- 1/2 lb shrimp, peeled and deveined
- 1 avocado, diced
- 1 cup cherry tomatoes, halved
- 2 cups mixed greens
- 1 tablespoon olive oil
- 1 tablespoon balsamic vinegar
- Salt and pepper to taste

Benefits of Omega-3 Fatty Acids: Shrimp is a good source of omega-3 fatty acids, which support hormone balance and may help reduce inflammation associated with PCOS

Directions

- Warm up olive oil in a skillet on medium heat.
- Add shrimp to the skillet and cook for 2-3 minutes on each side until pink and cooked through.
- In a large bowl, combine mixed greens, cherry tomatoes, and diced avocado.
- Drizzle balsamic vinegar over the salad and toss to coat.
- Divide the salad between two plates and top with cooked shrimp.
- Add salt and pepper according to taste before serving.

Tuna Stuffed Bell Peppers

| Servings: 4 | Prep time: 15 min | Cook time: 25 min | Total time: 40 min |

Nutrition per Serving: Calories: 220, Protein: 30g, Sodium: 450mg, Carbohydrates: 15g, Fat: 5g

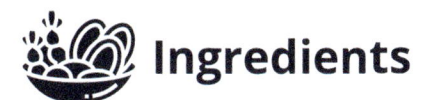

Ingredients

- 4 bell peppers, cut in half with seeds removed
- 2 cans of tuna, each 5 ounces, drained
- 1/2 cup diced celery
- 1/4 cup diced red onion
- 1/4 cup plain Greek yogurt
- 1 tablespoon Dijon mustard
- 1 tablespoon lemon juice
- 1 teaspoon dried dill
- Salt and pepper to taste
- Optional: Shredded cheese for topping

Benefits of Omega-3 Fatty Acids: Tuna is rich in omega-3 fatty acids, which can help reduce inflammation and support hormone balance in women with PCOS.

Directions

- Preheat the oven to 375°F (190°C)
- Place bell pepper halves in a baking dish, cut side up
- In a large bowl, mix together drained tuna, diced celery, diced red onion, Greek yogurt, Dijon mustard, lemon juice, and dried dill
- Season with salt and pepper to taste
- Spoon the tuna mixture evenly into each bell pepper half
- If you prefer, add shredded cheese on top of each stuffed pepper
- Cover the baking dish with foil and bake for 20-25 minutes until peppers are tender
- Unwrap the foil, place in oven, and bake for an extra 5 minutes until cheese is melted and bubbling
- Serve hot and enjoy!

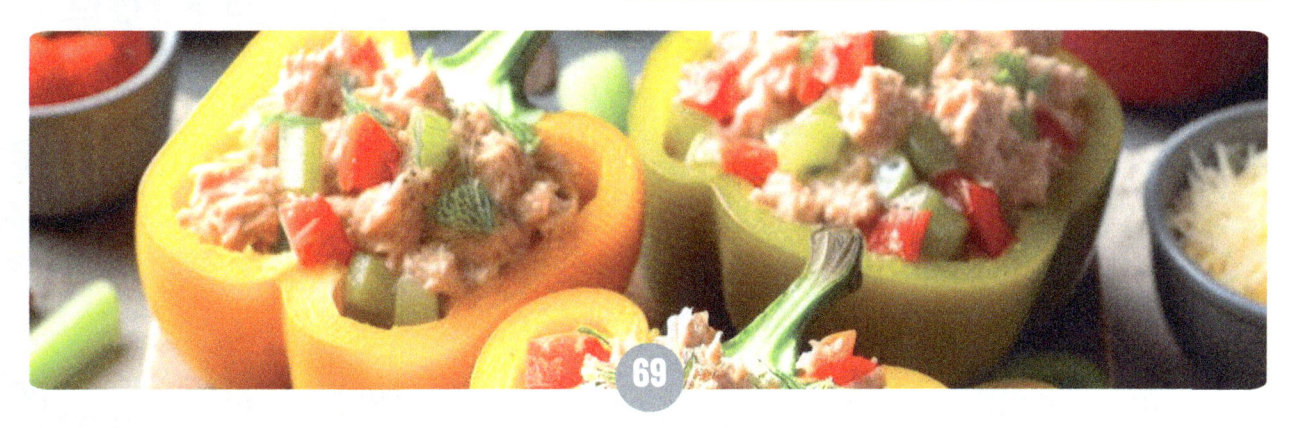

Grilled Lemon Garlic Swordfish

Servings: 4	Prep time: 10 min	Cook time: 10 min	Total time: 20 min

<u>Nutrition per Serving:</u> Calories: 250, Protein: 32g, Sodium: 200mg, Carbohydrates: 2g, Fat: 12g

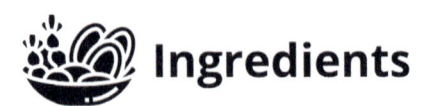

Ingredients

- 4 swordfish steaks
- 2 cloves garlic, minced
- 2 tablespoons olive oil
- 1 lemon, juiced and zested
- 1 teaspoon dried oregano
- Salt and pepper to taste
- Fresh parsley for garnish

Benefits of Omega-3 Fatty Acids: Swordfish is a rich source of omega-3 fatty acids, which are known for their anti-inflammatory properties and ability to support hormone balance in women with PCOS.

Directions

- Preheat grill to medium-high heat
- Combine minced garlic, olive oil, lemon juice, lemon zest, and dried oregano in a small bowl to create the marinade
- Then, season both sides of the swordfish steaks with salt and pepper
- Brush the marinade over the swordfish steaks, coating them evenly
- Place swordfish steaks on the preheated grill and cook for 4-5 minutes on each side until fish is opaque and flakes easily with a fork
- Remove swordfish from the grill and garnish with fresh parsley before serving

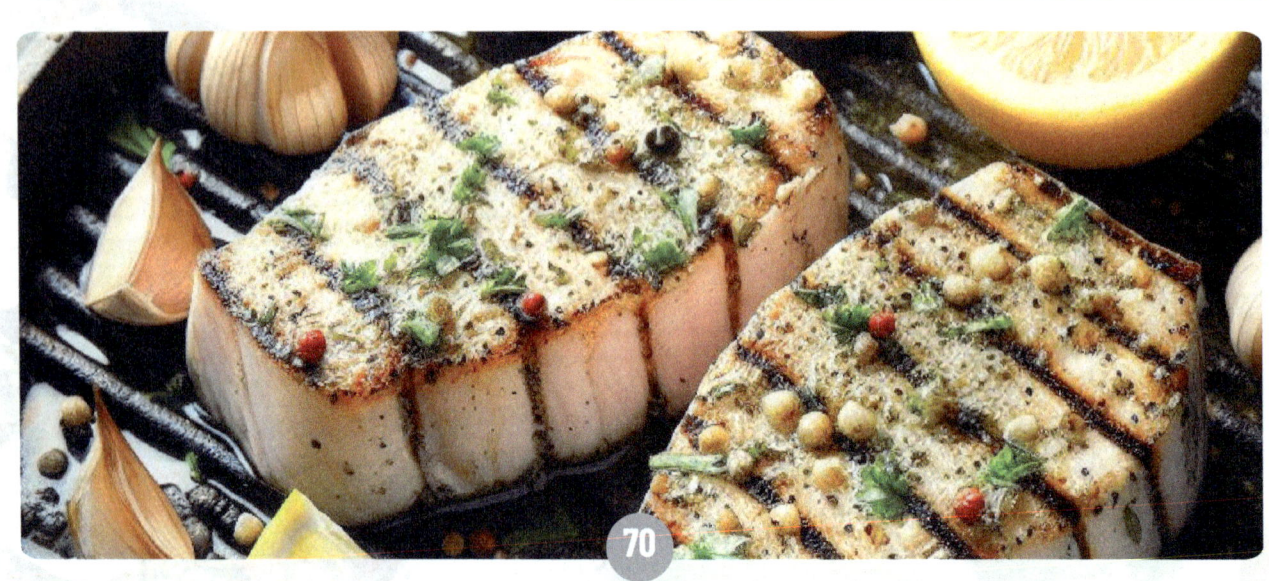

Quick and Easy Seafood Suppers

Lemon Garlic Shrimp Stir-Fry

| Servings: 4 | Prep time: 10 min | Cook time: 10 min | Total time: 20 min |

Nutrition per Serving: Calories: 180, Protein: 20g, Carbohydrates: 8g, Fat: 8g, Fiber: 2g

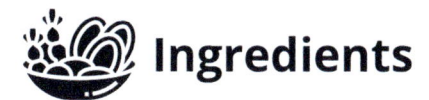

Ingredients

- 1 pound shrimp, peeled and deveined
- 2 tablespoons olive oil
- 4 cloves garlic, minced
- 1 bell pepper, thinly sliced
- 1 cup broccoli florets
- 1 tablespoon low-sodium soy sauce (or tamari for gluten-free)
- Juice of 1 lemon
- Salt and pepper to taste
- Already cooked brown rice or quinoa, for serving

Directions

- In a sizable skillet, warm olive oil over medium-high heat.
- Add minced garlic to the skillet and sauté for 1 minute until fragrant.
- Add shrimp to the skillet and cook for 2-3 minutes until pink and opaque.
- Stir in bell pepper and broccoli florets, and cook for an additional 3-4 minutes until vegetables are tender-crisp.
- Drizzle soy sauce and lemon juice over the shrimp and vegetables, and toss to coat evenly.
- Season with salt and pepper to taste.
- Serve the stir-fry hot over cooked brown rice or quinoa.

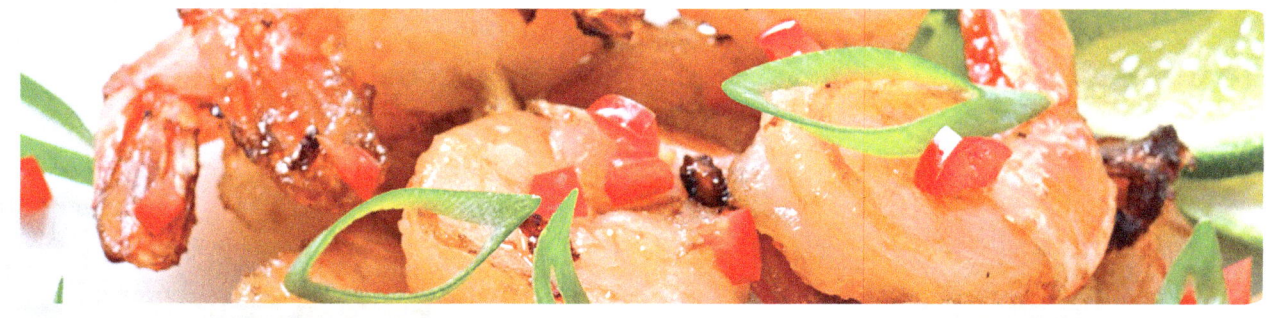

Pairing Suggestion: Enjoy this flavorful stir-fry with hormone-regulating ingredients like bell peppers and broccoli, which add a burst of color and nutrients to your meal

Herb-Crusted Baked Cod

| Servings: 4 | Prep time: 10 min | Cook time: 15 min | Total time: 25 min |

Nutrition per Serving: Calories: 200, Protein: 30g, Sodium: 100mg, Carbohydrates: 1g, Fat: 8g

Ingredients

- 4 cod fillets
- 2 tablespoons olive oil
- 1 tablespoon fresh parsley, chopped
- 1 tablespoon fresh dill, chopped
- 1 teaspoon lemon zest
- 2 cloves garlic, minced
- Salt and pepper to taste
- Lemon wedges, for serving

Pairing Suggestion: Pair this herb-crusted cod with a side of hormone-regulating vegetables like asparagus or spinach for a well-rounded and nutritious meal.

Directions

- Preheat the oven to 400°F (200°C).
- Arrange cod fillets on a baking sheet covered with parchment paper.
- In a small bowl, combine olive oil, chopped parsley, chopped dill, lemon zest, minced garlic, salt, and pepper to make the herb crust.
- Spread the herb crust evenly over the top of each cod fillet.
- Bake for 12-15 minutes until fish is cooked through and flakes easily with a fork.
- Serve hot with lemon wedges on the side.

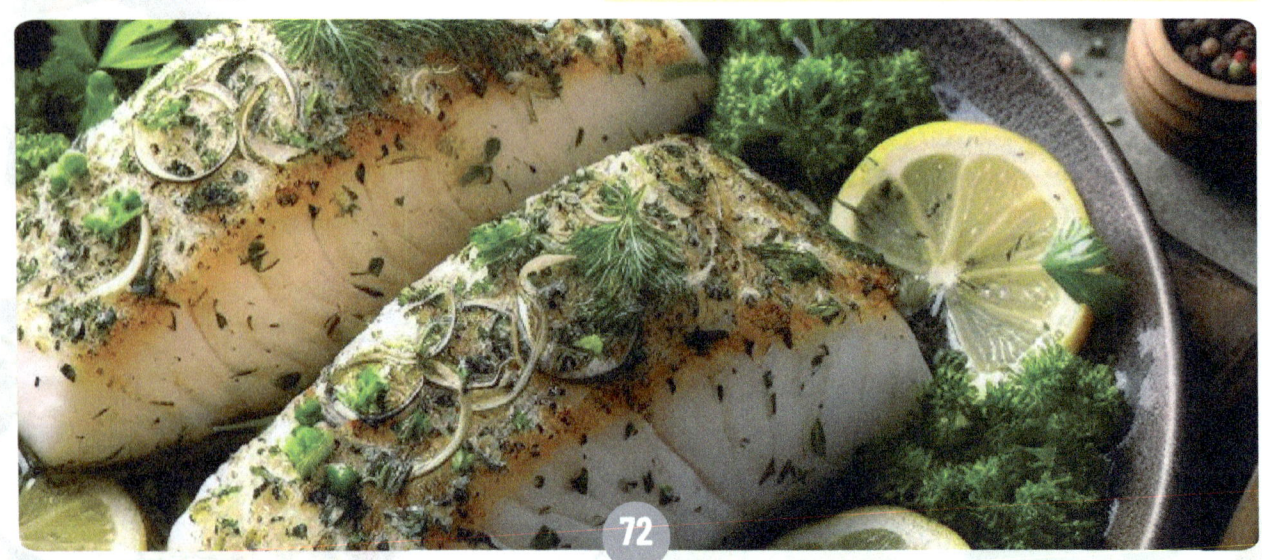

Coconut Curry Shrimp

| Servings: 4 | Prep time: 15 min | Cook time: 15 min | Total time: 30 min |

Nutrition per Serving: Calories: 280, Protein: 18g, Carbohydrates: 9g, Fat: 20g, Fiber: 2g

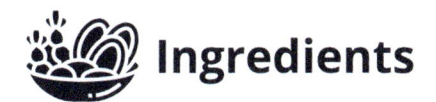

Ingredients

- 1 pound shrimp, peeled and deveined
- 1 tablespoon coconut oil
- 1 onion, diced
- 2 cloves garlic, minced
- 1 tablespoon grated ginger
- 1 red bell pepper, sliced
- 1 cup broccoli florets
- 2 tablespoons red curry paste
- 1 can (14 oz) coconut milk
- 1 tablespoon fish sauce
- 1 tablespoon lime juice
- Fresh cilantro, for garnish
- Cooked brown rice, for serving

Pairing Suggestion: Enjoy this aromatic coconut curry shrimp with a side of hormone-balancing leafy greens like kale or Swiss chard for a satisfying and nutritious meal.

Directions

- On medium heat, warm coconut oil in a large skillet.
- Add diced onion, minced garlic, and grated ginger to the skillet. Sauté until fragrant, about 2 minutes.
- Include sliced red bell pepper and broccoli florets in the skillet.. Cook for another 3-4 minutes until vegetables are slightly softened.
- Push the vegetables to the side of the skillet and add the shrimp. Cook for 2-3 minutes on each side until both sides are pink and fully cooked.
- Stir in red curry paste, coconut milk, fish sauce, and lime juice. Bring the mixture to a simmer and cook for 5 minutes until the sauce thickens slightly.
- Serve the coconut curry shrimp hot over cooked brown rice.
- Garnish with fresh cilantro before serving.

Lemon Herb Grilled Salmon

Servings: 4	Prep time: 10 min	Cook time: 10 min	Total time: 20 min

Nutrition per Serving: Calories: 300, Protein: 25g, Carbohydrates: 1g, Fat: 20g, Sodium: 100mg

Ingredients

- 4 salmon fillets
- 2 tablespoons olive oil
- 1 tablespoon fresh lemon juice
- 2 cloves garlic, minced
- 1 teaspoon dried oregano
- 1 teaspoon dried thyme
- Salt and pepper to taste
- Lemon slices, for garnish

Directions

- Preheat grill to medium-high heat.
- In a small bowl, whisk together olive oil, lemon juice, minced garlic, dried oregano, dried thyme, salt, and pepper to make the marinade.
- Place salmon fillets on a plate and brush both sides with the marinade.
- Grill salmon fillets for 4-5 minutes on each side until cooked through and grill marks appear.
- Remove salmon from the grill and garnish with lemon slices before serving.
- Serve hot alongside your favorite hormone-regulating vegetables or whole grains.

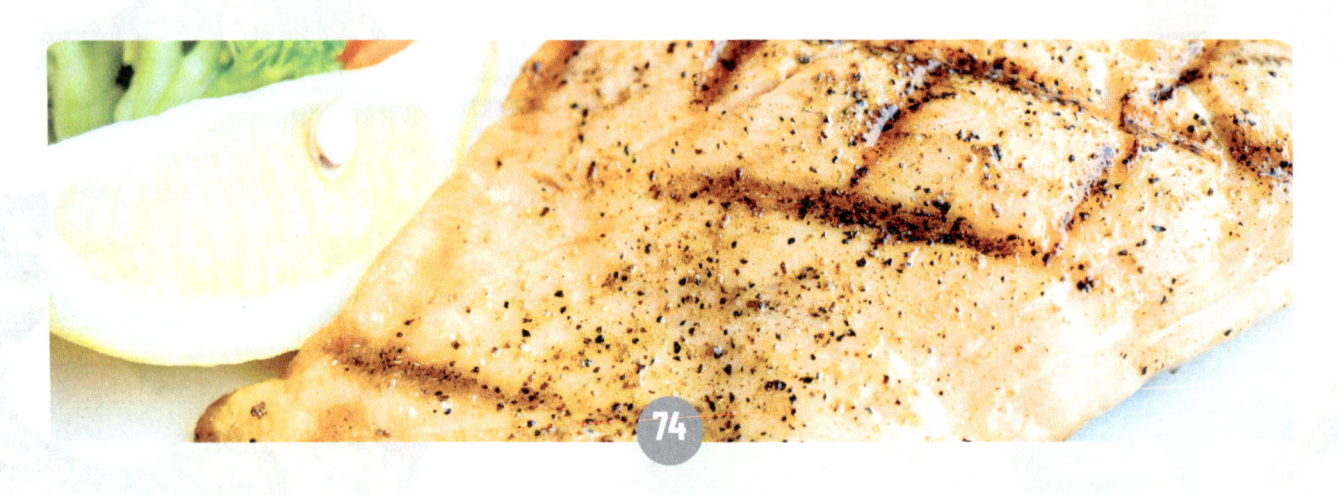

Pairing Suggestion: Pair this lemon herb grilled salmon with hormone-regulating vegetables like zucchini or Brussels sprouts for a balanced and flavorful meal.

Grilled Salmon with Lemon Dill Marinade

Servings: 4,   Prep Time: 10 min   Cook Time: 10 min,   Total Time: 20 min

Nutrition per Serving: Calories: 280, Protein: 26g, Sodium: 90mg, Carbohydrates: 1g, Fat: 18g

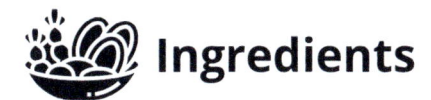

Ingredients

- 4 salmon fillets
- 2 tablespoons olive oil
- Juice of 1 lemon
- Zest of 1 lemon
- 2 cloves garlic, minced
- 1 tablespoon fresh dill, chopped
- Salt and pepper to taste
- Lemon wedges for serving

Healthy Cooking Tip: Grilling salmon helps retain its natural moisture and flavor while adding a delicious smoky char.

Directions

- Preheat grill to medium-high heat.
- In a small bowl, whisk together olive oil, lemon juice, lemon zest, minced garlic, and chopped dill.
- Season salmon fillets with salt and pepper, then brush both sides with the lemon dill marinade.
- Grill salmon fillets for 4-5 minutes on each side, or until fish is cooked through and flakes easily with a fork.
- Serve hot with lemon wedges for an extra burst of flavor.

Baked Cod with Herbed Panko Crust

Servings: 4,   Prep Time: 15 min   Cook Time: 15 min,   Total Time: 30 min

Nutrition per Serving: Calories: 220, Protein: 30g, Sodium: 200mg, Carbohydrates: 9g, Fat: 6g

Ingredients

- 4 cod fillets
- 1 tablespoon olive oil
- 1/2 cup panko breadcrumbs
- 1 tablespoon fresh parsley, chopped
- 1 tablespoon fresh dill, chopped
- 1 teaspoon lemon zest
- 1 teaspoon garlic powder
- Salt and pepper to taste
- Lemon wedges for serving

Healthy Cooking Tip: Baking cod with a herbed panko crust creates a crispy, flavorful coating without excess oil or calories.

Directions

- Preheat oven to 400°F (200°C).
- Arrange cod fillets on a baking sheet covered with parchment paper.
- In a small bowl, mix together panko breadcrumbs, chopped parsley, chopped dill, lemon zest, garlic powder, salt, and pepper.
- Brush cod fillets with olive oil, then press the breadcrumb mixture onto the top of each fillet.
- Bake in the oven for 12-15 minutes, or until the fish becomes opaque and easily flakes apart when pierced with a fork.
- Serve hot with lemon wedges on the side.

Grilled Halibut with Citrus Herb Marinade

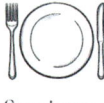

| Servings: 4 | Prep time: 15 min | Cook time: 10 min | Total time: 25 min |

Nutrition per Serving: Calories: 240, Protein: 35g, Carbohydrates: 3g, Fat: 10g, Sodium: 150mg

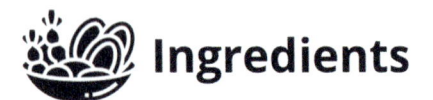

Ingredients

- 4 halibut fillets
- 2 tablespoons olive oil
- Juice of 1 lemon
- Juice of 1 orange
- 2 cloves garlic, minced
- 1 tablespoon fresh thyme, chopped
- 1 tablespoon fresh parsley, chopped
- Salt and pepper to taste
- Lemon wedges for serving

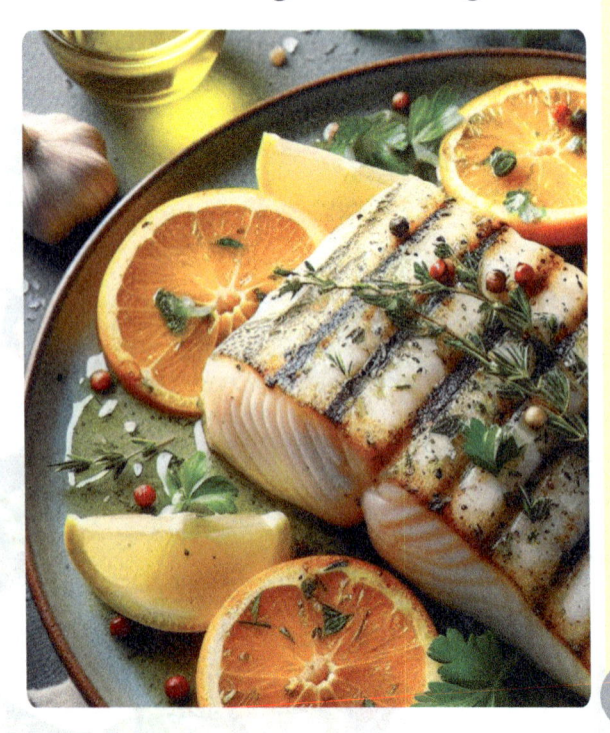

Directions

- In a small bowl, whisk together olive oil, lemon juice, orange juice, minced garlic, chopped thyme, and chopped parsley.
- Season halibut fillets with salt and pepper, then place them in a shallow dish or resealable plastic bag.
- Pour the citrus herb marinade over the halibut, ensuring it is evenly coated.
- Allow to marinate in the refrigerator for a minimum of 30 minutes, or for up to 2 hours.
- Preheat grill to medium-high heat. Remove halibut from marinade and discard excess marinade.
- Grill halibut fillets for 4-5 minutes on each side, or until fish is opaque and flakes easily with a fork.
- Serve hot with lemon wedges on the side.

Healthy Cooking Tip: Grilling halibut with a citrus herb marinade adds bright, fresh flavors while keeping the fish tender and juicy.

BONUS

PCOS
DIET COOKBOOK

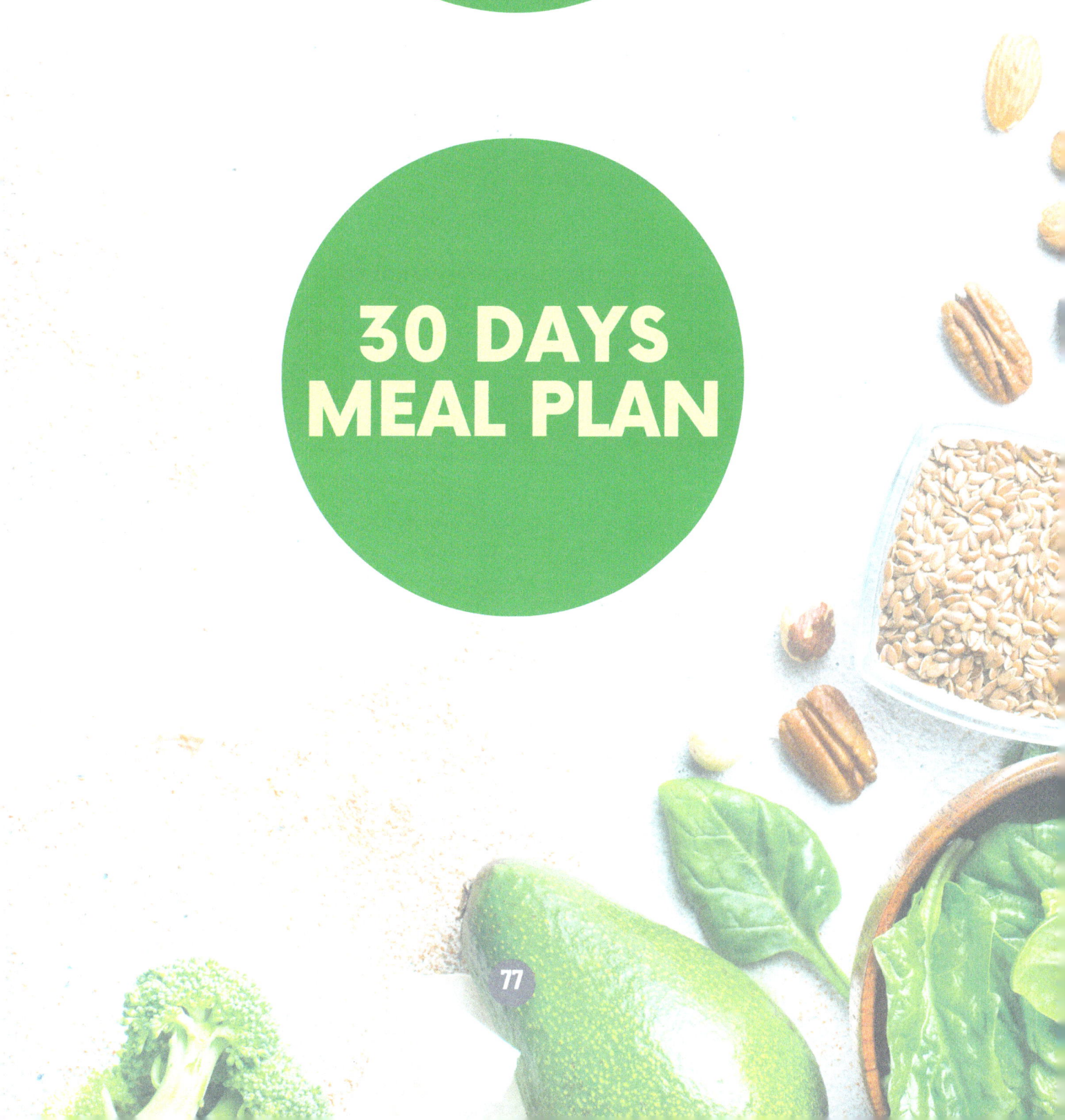

30 DAYS MEAL PLAN

PCOS-FRIENDLY MEALS

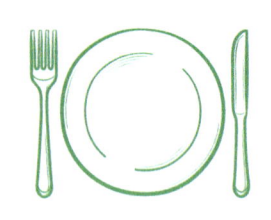

Breakfast:
Berry Blast Smoothie
Green Goddess Shake
Tropical Paradise Smoothie
Peanut Butter Power Shake
Vanilla Almond Overnight Oats
Creamy Coconut Chia Pudding
Spinach and Feta Omelet
Veggie-Packed Breakfast Scramble

Lunch:
Hormone-Balancing Quinoa Power Bowl
Quinoa Salad with Citrus Dressing
Lentil and Sweet Potato Stew
Lentil and Spinach Soup
Chickpea and Avocado Wrap
Turkey and Hummus Wrap

Dinner:
Wholesome One-Pot Quinoa Primavera
Hearty Lentil and Vegetable Stew
Lemon Herb Salmon and Vegetable Medley
Vibrant Mediterranean Chicken and Veggie Delight
Savory Shrimp Stir-Fry
Flavorful Tofu and Vegetable Stir-Fry

Dessert:
Lemon-Kissed Cinnamon Baked Apples
Veggie and Hummus Snack Packs
Chocolate Chip Banana Bread Bars
Raspberry Chia Seed Pudding Parfaits
Protein-Packed Berry Bliss Nice Cream
Superfood Spinach-Berry Popsicles

Beverages:
Hormone Harmony Blend
Insulin Support Blend
Anti-inflammatory Elixir
Digestive Ease Blend
Stress Relief Soother
Liver Love Infusion
Berry Blast Smoothie Booster
Green Goddess Juice Booster
Tropical Turmeric Smoothie Booster
Creamy Cocoa Protein Shake
Golden Glow Turmeric Latte
Berry Beet Detox Juice

Vegetarian and vegan Entrées:
Quinoa Stuffed Bell Peppers
Lentil and Vegetable Stir-Fry
Chickpea and Vegetable Curry
Eggplant and Lentil Moussaka
Spinach and Chickpea Curry
Mushroom and Lentil Shepherd's Pie
Mediterranean Farro Salad
Vegetable Stir-Fry with Brown Rice
Vegetable and Chickpea Coconut Curry
Creamy Avocado Pasta
Coconut Curry Lentil Soup
Dairy-Free Pesto Zoodles
Dairy-Free Spinach and Mushroom Risotto

Fish and seafood Entrées:
Salmon with Lemon Dill Sauce
Miso Glazed Cod
Shrimp and Avocado Salad
Tuna Stuffed Bell Peppers
Grilled Lemon Garlic Swordfish
Lemon Garlic Shrimp Stir-Fry
Herb-Crusted Baked Cod
Coconut Curry Shrimp
Lemon Herb Grilled Salmon
Grilled Salmon with Lemon Dill Marinade
Grilled Halibut with Citrus Herb Marinade

WEEK ONE MEAL PLAN

Day 1: • Breakfast: Creamy Avocado Pasta • Lunch: Coconut Curry Lentil Soup • Dinner: Dairy-Free Pesto Zoodles • Dessert: Lemon-Kissed Cinnamon Baked Apples	**MONDAY**
Day 2: • Breakfast: Coconut Chia Pudding • Lunch: Hormone-Balancing Quinoa Power Bowl • Dinner: Wholesome One-Pot Quinoa Primavera • Dessert: Chocolate Chip Banana Bread Bars	**TUESDAY**
Day 3: • Breakfast: Berry Blast Smoothie • Lunch: Dairy-Free Spinach and Mushroom Risotto • Dinner: Hearty Lentil and Vegetable Stew • Dessert: Raspberry Chia Seed Pudding Parfaits	**WEDNESDAY**
Day 4: • Breakfast: Green Goddess Shake • Lunch: Lentil and Vegetable Stir-Fry • Dinner: Lemon Herb Salmon and Vegetable Medley • Dessert: Superfood Spinach-Berry Popsicles	**THURSDAY**
Day 5: • Breakfast: Tropical Paradise Smoothie • Lunch: Mediterranean Chickpea Salad • Dinner: Coconut Curry Shrimp • Dessert: Veggie and Hummus Snack Packs	**FRIDAY**
Day 6: • Breakfast: Peanut Butter Power Shake • Lunch: Lentil and Spinach Soup • Dinner: Vibrant Mediterranean Chicken and Veggie Delight • Dessert: Lemon-Kissed Cinnamon Baked Apples	**SATURDAY**
Day 7: • Breakfast: Vanilla Almond Overnight Oats • Lunch: Chickpea and Avocado Wrap • Dinner: Savory Shrimp Stir-Fry • Dessert: Protein-Packed Berry Bliss Nice Cream	**SUNDAY**

WEEK TWO MEAL PLAN

Day 8: • Breakfast: Creamy Coconut Chia Pudding • Lunch: Turkey and Hummus Wrap • Dinner: Flavorful Tofu and Vegetable Stir-Fry • Dessert: Chocolate Chip Banana Bread Bars	**MONDAY**
Day 9: • Breakfast: Spinach and Feta Omelet • Lunch: Hormone-Balancing Quinoa Power Bowl • Dinner: Wholesome One-Pot Quinoa Primavera • Dessert: Lemon-Kissed Cinnamon Baked Apples	**TUESDAY**
Day 10: • Breakfast: Berry Blast Smoothie • Lunch: Quinoa Salad with Citrus Dressing • Dinner: Hearty Lentil and Vegetable Stew • Dessert: Superfood Spinach-Berry Popsicles	**WEDNESDAY**
Day 11: • Breakfast: Green Goddess Shake • Lunch: Lentil and Sweet Potato Stew • Dinner: Lemon Herb Salmon and Vegetable Medley • Dessert: Lemon-Kissed Cinnamon Baked Apples	**THURSDAY**
Day 12: • Breakfast: Tropical Paradise Smoothie • Lunch: Lentil and Spinach Soup • Dinner: Vibrant Mediterranean Chicken and Veggie Delight • Dessert: Chocolate Chip Banana Bread Bars	**FRIDAY**
Day 13: • Breakfast: Peanut Butter Power Shake • Lunch: Chickpea and Avocado Wrap • Dinner: Savory Shrimp Stir-Fry • Dessert: Raspberry Chia Seed Pudding Parfaits	**SATURDAY**
Day 14: • Breakfast: Vanilla Almond Overnight Oats • Lunch: Turkey and Hummus Wrap • Dinner: Flavorful Tofu and Vegetable Stir-Fry • Dessert: Veggie and Hummus Snack Packs	**SUNDAY**

WEEK THREE MEAL PLAN

MONDAY
Day 15:
- Breakfast: Tropical Paradise Smoothie
- Lunch: Chickpea and Vegetable Curry (Vegan)
- Dinner: Grilled Lemon Garlic Swordfish
- Dessert: Chocolate Chip Banana Bread Bars

TUESDAY
Day 16:
- Breakfast: Peanut Butter Power Shake
- Lunch: Lentil and Vegetable Stir-Fry (Vegan)
- Dinner: Lemon Herb Grilled Salmon
- Dessert: Lemon-Kissed Cinnamon Baked Apples

WEDNESDAY
Day 17:
- Breakfast: Vanilla Almond Overnight Oats
- Lunch: Mediterranean Farro Salad (Vegetarian)
- Dinner: Chickpea and Vegetable Curry (Vegan)
- Dessert: Chocolate Chip Banana Bread Bars

THURSDAY
Day 18:
- Breakfast: Creamy Coconut Chia Pudding
- Lunch: Vegetable Stir-Fry with Brown Rice (Vegan)
- Dinner: Coconut Curry Shrimpe
- Dessert: Lemon-Kissed Cinnamon Baked Apples

FRIDAY
Day 19:
- Breakfast: Berry Blast Smoothie
- Lunch: Lentil and Vegetable Stir-Fry (Vegan)
- Dinner: Lemon Herb Grilled Salmon
- Dessert: Chocolate Chip Banana Bread Bars

SATURDAY
Day 20:
- Breakfast: Green Goddess Shake
- Lunch: Quinoa Salad with Citrus Dressing (Vegetarian)
- Dinner: Grilled Halibut with Citrus Herb Marinade
- Dessert: Superfood Spinach-Berry Popsicles

SUNDAY
Day 21:
- Breakfast: Peanut Butter Power Shake
- Lunch: Lentil and Vegetable Stir-Fry (Vegan)
- Dinner: Lemon Herb Grilled Salmon
- Dessert: Lemon-Kissed Cinnamon Baked Apples

WEEK FOUR MEAL PLAN

Day 22: • Breakfast: Vanilla Almond Overnight Oats • Lunch: Chickpea and Vegetable Curry (Vegan) • Dinner: Lemon Herb Grilled Salmon • Dessert: Chocolate Chip Banana Bread Bars	**MONDAY**
Day 23: • Breakfast: Creamy Coconut Chia Pudding • Lunch: Quinoa Stuffed Bell Peppers (Vegetarian) • Dinner: Grilled Lemon Garlic Swordfish • Dessert: Raspberry Chia Seed Pudding Parfaits	**TUESDAY**
Day 24: • Breakfast: Berry Blast Smoothie • Lunch: Lentil and Spinach Soup (Vegan) • Dinner: Quinoa Stuffed Bell Peppers (Vegetarian) • Dessert: Veggie and Hummus Snack Packs	**WEDNESDAY**
Day 25: • Breakfast: Dairy-Free Peach Pie Smoothie Bowl • Lunch: Lentil and Roasted Vegetable Salad with Balsamic Vinaigrette • Dinner: Vegan Coconut Curry Lentil Soup	**THURSDAY**
Day 26: • Breakfast: Tropical Paradise Smoothie • Lunch: Chickpea and Vegetable Curry (Vegan) • Dinner: Grilled Lemon Garlic Swordfish • Dessert: Chocolate Chip Banana Bread Bars	**FRIDAY**
Day 27: • Breakfast: Peanut Butter Power Shake • Lunch: Lentil and Vegetable Stir-Fry (Vegan) • Dinner: Lemon Herb Grilled Salmon • Dessert: Lemon-Kissed Cinnamon Baked Apples	**SATURDAY**
Day 28: • Breakfast: Vanilla Almond Overnight Oats • Lunch: Mediterranean Farro Salad (Vegetarian) • Dinner: Chickpea and Vegetable Curry (Vegan) • Dessert: Chocolate Chip Banana Bread Bars	**SUNDAY**

Day 29: • Breakfast: Berry Blast Smoothie • Lunch: Lentil and Vegetable Stir-Fry (Vegan) • Dinner: Lemon Herb Grilled Salmon • Dessert: Chocolate Chip Banana Bread Bars	**WEEK FIVE MEAL PLAN** **MONDAY**
Day 30: • Breakfast: Green Goddess Shake • Lunch: Quinoa Salad with Citrus Dressing (Vegetarian) • Dinner: Grilled Halibut with Citrus Herb Marinade • Dessert: Superfood Spinach-Berry Popsicles	**TUESDAY**

Shopping List

Proteins:
- Salmon fillets
- Cod fillets
- Shrimp
- Tuna cans
- Eggs
- Tofu
- Lentils
- Chickpeas
- Chicken breast
- Beef (for some recipes)

Grains and Carbohydrates:
- Quinoa
- Farro
- Brown rice
- Whole grain bread
- Rolled oats
- Pasta (for some recipes)
- Sweet potatoes
- Potatoes
- Rice noodles

Fruits:
- Mixed berries (strawberries, blueberries, raspberries)
- Apples
- Bananas
- Lemons
- Oranges
- Mangoes
- Pineapples
- Peaches

Dairy and Non-Dairy Alternatives:
- Almond milk
- Coconut milk
- Hummus
- Coconut cream

Herbs and Spices:
- Dill
- Lemons
- Turmeric
- Cinnamon
- Garlic powder
- Ginger
- Paprika
- Cumin
- Coriander
- Oregano
- Basil
- Parsley
- Thyme
- Rosemary

Other Ingredients:
- Olive oil
- Coconut oil
- Peanut butter
- Chia seeds
- Flaxseeds
- Unsweetened cocoa powder
- Dark chocolate chips
- Maple syrup
- Honey
- Balsamic vinegar
- Apple cider vinegar
- Soy sauce
- Miso paste
- Vegetable broth
- Pesto sauce

Frozen Items:
- Mixed berries
- Spinach
- Assorted vegetables

Vegetables:
- Spinach
- Bell peppers
- Tomatoes
- Cucumbers
- Eggplants
- Mushrooms
- Zucchinis
- Lettuce
- Onions
- Garlic
- Assorted vegetables (carrots, broccoli, cauliflower, etc.)

Miscellaneous:
- Protein powder (optional)
- Assorted herbal teas

CONCLUSION

In conclusion, this cookbook is not just a compilation of recipes; it's a guide tailored specifically for women managing PCOS, offering a holistic approach to health and well-being. Through meticulously curated recipes and meal plans, we've strived to address the unique challenges faced by individuals with PCOS, from hormonal imbalances to dietary considerations.

With an emphasis on nutrient-rich ingredients, balanced meals, and flavorful combinations, this cookbook aims to empower you on your journey towards better health. Whether you're seeking to manage symptoms, support hormone balance, or simply adopt a healthier lifestyle, each recipe is thoughtfully crafted to provide nourishment and satisfaction.

Beyond the kitchen, this cookbook serves as a companion on your wellness journey, offering valuable insights, practical tips, and a sense of community. It's a reminder that you're not alone in your struggles, and that small, mindful changes can make a significant difference in your quality of life.

As you embark on this culinary adventure, remember that nourishing your body is an act of self-love. Celebrate every step forward, embrace the journey, and savor the delicious flavors that await. You have the power to take control of your health and thrive, one nourishing meal at a time.

Here's to your health, happiness, and the boundless possibilities that lie ahead. Cheers to the vibrant, empowered woman you are, and may this cookbook be a source of inspiration and empowerment on your path to wellness.

ABOUT THE AUTHOR

Emily Lexie is a dedicated holistic nutritionist and women's health advocate with a passion for empowering individuals with PCOS to take control of their health and well-being. Drawing from her personal journey and professional expertise, Emily has devoted her career to empowering women to take control of their health and wellness.

With a background in nutritional science and extensive experience in PCOS management, Emily understands the complexities of the condition and the unique challenges it presents. Her own journey with PCOS has inspired her to look deeper into the realms of holistic health, seeking sustainable solutions rooted in nutrition, lifestyle, and self-care.

Through her work and personal experiences, Emily has developed a deep understanding of the importance of nutrition in managing PCOS symptoms. Her commitment to supporting women on their journey to hormonal balance is evident in her book, "The PCOS Diet Cookbook: The Complete Guide with Flavorful Recipes to Manage Polycystic Ovary Syndrome, Regulate your Hormones, and Improve Fertility."

Emily's mission is to educate, inspire, and uplift individuals with PCOS, providing them with the tools, support, and encouragement they need to live vibrant, fulfilling lives. Through her work, Emily aims to encourage the development of a community of empowerment, resilience, and hope, where every woman with PCOS can find strength, healing, and transformation.

Expressing my heartfelt gratitude

I am deeply grateful for your decision to purchase this Cookbook tailored specifically for women managing PCOS symptoms. I'm thrilled to hear about your experience with these recipes and how they've positively impacted your health journey

As an independent publisher, your voice and feedback hold immense value. They not only inspire me to continually refine my work but also guide others on their path toward being able to balance their hormones and manage their PCOS symptoms as well. If you found value in this Diet Cookbook, I kindly request that you consider leaving a review on Amazon.

Your insights and experiences can make a profound difference in both supporting my mission and assisting countless others in benefiting from this Cookbook.

From the depths of my heart, I extend my sincere gratitude for joining me on this journey. Your support fuels my passion and purpose.

With warm regards,

Emily Lexie

PCOS DIET COOKBOOK

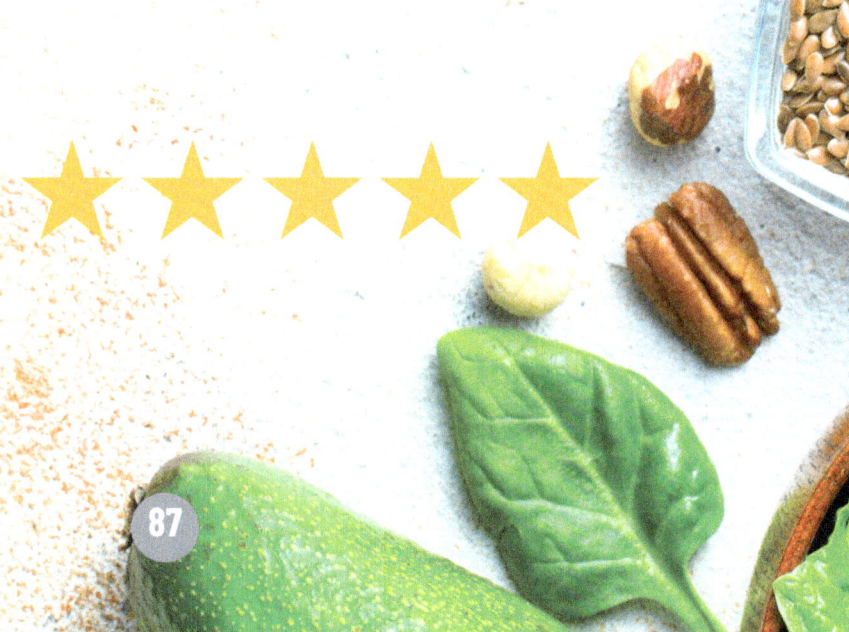

APPENDIX

The Glycemic Index And Glycemic Load Food List

Below is a comprehensive list categorizing common carbohydrates based on their glycemic index (GI) and glycemic load (GL), which indicate their impact on blood glucose levels. Foods are scored between 0 and 100 on the GI scale, with ideal options falling within the range of 55 to 69. However, it's crucial to prioritize the glycemic load of a food, which considers the quantity of carbohydrates per serving. Optimal choices typically boast low (under 10) or moderate (between 10 and 20) glycemic loads.

FOOD	GLYCEMIC INDEX	SERVING SIZE grams, unless noted othewise	GLYCEMIC LOAD per serving
Bakery Products			
Bagel, white	72	70	25
Baguette, white	95	30	15
Barley bread	34	30	7
Corn tortilla	52	50	12
Croissant	67	57	17
Doughnut	76	47	17
Pita bread	68	30	10
Sourdough rye	48	30	6
Soya and linseed bread	36	30	3

Sponge cake	46	63	17
Wheat tortilla	30	50	8
White wheat flour bread	71	30	10
Whole-wheat bread	71	30	9

Beverages

Apple juice, unsweetened	44	250 mL	30
Coca-Cola	63	250 mL	16
Gatorade	78	250 mL	12
Lucozade	95	250 mL	40
Orange juice, unsweetened	50	250 mL	12
Tomato juice, canned	38	250 mL	4

Breakfast Cereals

All-Bran	55	30	12
Cocoa Krispies	77	30	20
Cornflakes	93	30	23
Muesli, average	66	30	16

Oatmeal, average	55	50	13
Special K	69	30	14

Dairy

Ice cream, regular	57	50	6
Milk, full-fat	41	250 mL	5
Milk, skim	32	250 mL	4
Reduced-fat yogurt with fruit	33	200	11

Fruits

Apple	39	120	6
Banana, ripe	62	120	16
Cherries	22	120	3
Dates, dried	42	60	18
Grapefruit	25	120	3
Grapes	59	120	11
Mango	41	120	8
Orange	40	120	4

Peach	42	120	5
Pear	38	120	4
Pineapple	51	120	8
Raisins	64	60	28
Strawberries	40	120	1
Watermelon	72	120	4

Grains

Brown Rice	50	150	16
Buckwheat	45	150	13
Bulgur	30	50	11
Corn on the cob	60	150	20
Couscous	65	150	9
Fettuccini, average	32	180	15
Gnocchi	68	180	33
Macaroni, average	47	180	23
Quinoa	53	150	13

Spaghetti, white	46	180	22
Spaghetti, whole-wheat	42	180	26
Vermicelli noodles	35	180	16
White rice	89	150	43

Legumes

Baked beans	40	150	6
Black beans	30	150	7
Butter beans	36	150	8
Chickpeas	10	150	3
Kidney beans	29	150	7
Lentils	29	150	5
Navy beans	31	150	9
Soy beans	50	150	1

Snack Foods

Cashews, salted	27	50	3
Corn chips, plain, salted	42	50	11

Fruit Roll-Ups	99	30	24
Graham crackers	74	25	14
Honey	61	25	12
Hummus	6	30	0
M&M's, peanut	33	30	6
Microwave popcorn, plain	55	20	6
Muesli bar	61	30	13
Nutella	33	20	4
Peanuts	7	50	0
Potato chips, average	51	50	12
Pretzels	83	30	16
Rice cakes	82	25	17
Rye crisps	64	25	11
Shortbread	64	25	10
Vanilla wafers	77	25	14
Walnuts	15	28	0

Vegetables			
Beets	64	80	4
Carrot	35	80	2
Green peas	51	80	4
Parsnip	52	80	4
Sweet potato, average	70	150	22
White potato, boiled	81	150	22
Yam	54	150	20

Sources: Harvard Health Publications (www.health.harvard.edu/healthyeating/glycemic_index_and_glycemic_load_for_100_foods) Mendosa.com (www.mendosa.com/gilists.htm).

Printed in Great Britain
by Amazon